all-day energy

100 ways to boost your energy...now!

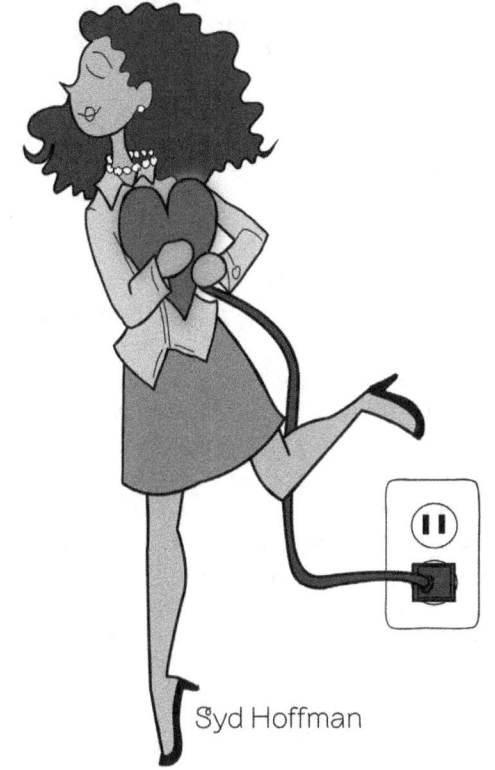

Syd Hoffman

All-Day Energy
100 ways to boost your energy … now!
By Syd Hoffman

ISBN-13: 978-1470191689
LOC: 2012906250

For information:
www.SydHoffman.com

Dedication

This book is dedicated to my beautiful mom, Fabulous Florence. Thanks for teaching me to eat well, play hard, and hug often. Your wisdom and kindness have touched my heart more than you'll ever know. I love you very much.

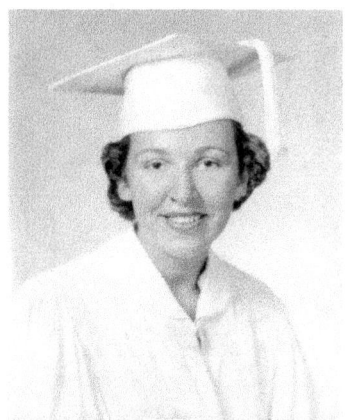

Fabulous Florence, June 1951

Introduction

*"How we spend our days is, of course,
how we spend our lives."*
—Annie Dillard, writer

All-Day Energy is based on one wonderful equation:
Happy Mind + Healthy Body = All-Day Energy

This book includes my favorite tips for maximizing
your energy. They are in no particular order.
Experiment. Explore. Reflect. And most
importantly ... have fun!

Please share your abundant energy with everyone
you meet along your journey!

Syd
xo.

Energizing Idea 1:
Sleep like a baby.

"May sleep envelop you as a bed sheet floating gently down, tickling your skin and removing every worry. Reminding you to consider only this moment."
—Jeb Dickerson

Many of us fall asleep with so much on our minds. Our brain is processing all the events of the day, planning what will be tomorrow, and stressing about what's not working perfectly. No wonder we wake up without feeling energized and renewed.

Wild idea!
Set aside a specific time (at least two hours before bedtime works best) to "download" any unfinished thoughts. Consider making tomorrow's to-do list, talking to a friend, writing in your journal, deciding on tasks to delegate, and/or jotting a note on your calendar. Be bold, ask the Universe for suggestions to find you tomorrow ... after your calm 7-8 hour rest. Go to sleep with a smile and the assurance that all is grand. Sleep like a baby.

More inspiration:
* www.SleepFoundation.org
* *Sound Sleep, Sound Mind: 7 Keys to Sleeping Through the Night* by Barry Krakow, M.D.

Affirmation:
I am thankful for all the good in my life. I look forward to waking up recharged and ready to go.

Energizing Idea 2:
Drink a glass of water.

"Water is the only drink for a wise man."
—Henry David Thoreau

Are you lacking the energy you need to get through your day? Is your thinking foggy and unclear? While a number of things can contribute to these symptoms, drinking plenty of water can often immediately enhance how you feel and function. Challenge yourself to drink more water throughout the day and notice the difference in how you feel. No other drink hydrates as well as water.

Things to consider:

- Every cell in your body needs water from head to toe. If you do not drink enough water, your brain cannot function, and you will likely experience a headache and other uncomfortable symptoms.
- Sometimes thirst masquerades itself as hunger. Increase your water intake and see if your cravings lessen. Add lemon, lime, cucumber, or a splash of juice for a different taste.

Enjoy this simple way to gain tremendous health benefits: weight loss, clarity, energy, healthy skin, and more.

More inspiration:
- www.AllAboutWater.org
- www.health-benefit-of-water.com

Affirmation:
I like the refreshing feeling that washes over my body as I drink a glass of water. Instant energy!

Energizing Idea 3:
Play with a sweet animal friend.

"Animals are such agreeable friends—they ask no questions; they pass no criticisms."
—George Eliot

There's something special about spending time with our pets. Researchers have shown pet owners have lower blood pressures and cholesterol levels. Caring for a pet boosts brain chemicals that reduce stress and make you feel happier. Pets provide unconditional love.

More inspiration:
* www.PetFinder.com
* Pets.WebMd.com/default.htm

Affirmation:
Spending time with animal friends brings me joy.

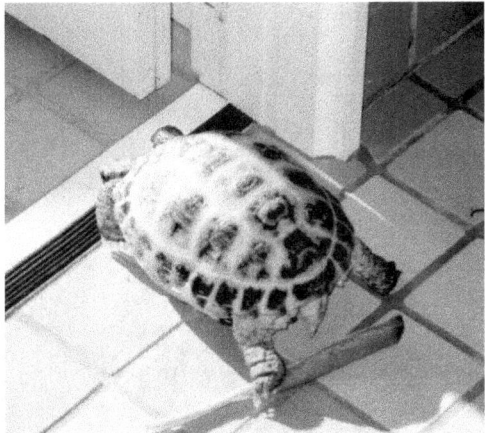

Rocky, our desert tortoise, "on the run" with a healthy green lettuce leaf.

Energizing Idea 4:
Avoid hidden calories in your salad.

"Salads can cost you upwards of 3,000 calories. Order your dressing on the side and dip your fork in it before taking each bite of salad."
—Amy Culver

The biggest culprits for turning a salad into a huge calorie meal are croutons, cheese, meats, and salad dressing. (Stick with lean turkey if you decide meat is a necessity.) I love to sprinkle a handful of raw unsalted nuts on my salad for protein. Add a few slices of fresh avocado for a yummy, healthy treat.

Wild idea!
Try what Dr. Oz does. In the morning or the night before, put nine walnuts in a little water (a snack bag or tiny container works well). At lunchtime, the liquid (water plus walnut oil) is your salad dressing! And the walnuts, sweeter after soaking, are perfect for topping your salad.

My ideal healthy salad …

_____
_____
_____
_____

More inspiration:
- *The Healthy Living Lifestyle* by Amy Culver
- *Prevention* magazine, a monthly publication

Affirmation:
I love creating a salad loaded with good health!

Energizing Idea 5:
Buy yourself fresh flowers.

*"When you have only two pennies left in the
world, buy a loaf of bread with one,
and a lily with the other."*
—Chinese Proverb

Treat yourself to the glorious aroma and vibrant
colors of fresh-cut flowers. Here are some thoughts
from my friends:

- "Flowers make an ordinary week feel like a
  special week!"
- "It's a surprise every time I see them on my
  kitchen table."
- "It's often foggy in San Francisco, flowers add
  a little sunshine."
- "I'm not waiting for someone to give me
  flowers … I'm contributing to my own
  happiness."
- "It makes me feel abundant!"
- "It turns my small apartment into a home."
- "Flowers remind me to slow down to enjoy
  the beauty in my life."

Affirmation:
I am worthy of all the beauty life has to offer.

To explore …

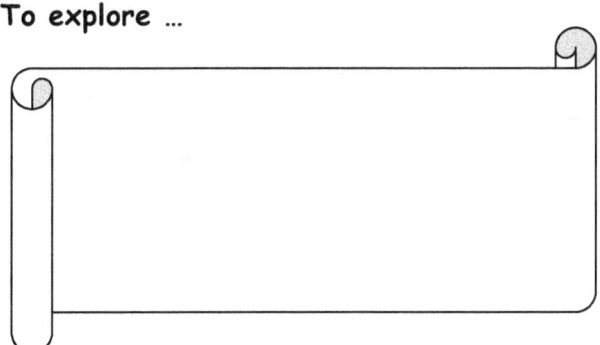

Energizing Idea 6:
Take a tea break.

*"There is no trouble so great or grave
that cannot be much diminished
by a nice cup of tea."*
—Bernard-Paul Heroux

A cup of herbal tea is an invitation to relax, reflect, and recharge in just a few minutes. For centuries, teas have been used for boosting energy, aiding healing, and cleansing.

- Pure herbal teas have no caffeine, artificial coloring, additives, or chemically produced flavors.
- Green tea has lots of disease-fighting antioxidants providing many health benefits. (If you need a little sweetness added, try stevia.)
- Mint tea eases digestive problems.
- Chamomile tea is useful for reducing stress and promoting restful sleep.

More inspiration:
- www.AllHerbalTea.com
- www.learn-about-tea.com
- *The New Tea Companion: A Guide to Teas Throughout the World* by Jane Pettigrew and Bruce Richardson

Affirmation:
I give myself permission to relax, reflect, and recharge.

Energizing Idea 7:
Yoga to the rescue.

"Yoga is invigoration in relaxation. Freedom in routine. Confidence through self-control. Energy within and energy without."
—Ymber Delecto

Yoga is excellent for improving your flexibility, balance, strength, mental clarity, and immune system. It provides tools to stay calm and present when life gets crazy. Yoga helps you sleep better.

More inspiration:

- *Yoga for Beginners: The Ultimate Guide to Getting Started* by Nicole Townsend
- *Yoga for Your Spiritual Muscles: A Complete Yoga Program to Strengthen Body and Spirit* by Rachael Schaeffer
- *Moving Toward Balance* by Rodney Yee with Nina Zolotow
- Yoga classes, DVDs, books, websites. Variety is fun!

Affirmation:

I calm my body by breathing deeply. I enjoy being flexible and balanced.

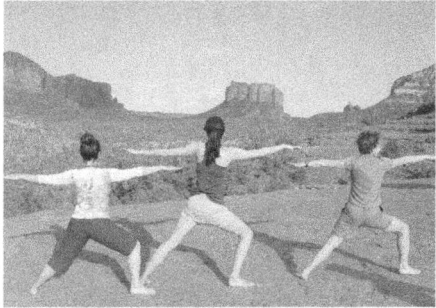

Sedona, AZ, May 2011

Energizing Idea 8:
Ask for help.

"You create your opportunities by
asking for them."
—Shakti Gawain

Somewhere along the way, we got it into our heads that asking for help shows weakness, insecurity, or stupidity. Let's flip that switch! Embrace the idea that asking for help is a sign of strength, confidence, and intelligence. Ask for what you need!

What I need help with right now ...

_____

_____

_____

_____

_____

_____

_____

More inspiration:

* *Creative Visualization* by Shakti Gawain
* *Ask and It Is Given: Learning to Manifest Your Desires* by Esther and Jerry Hicks

Affirmation:
I ask for what I need and I receive it. Life is grand!

Energizing Idea 9:
Single-task.

"In contrast to almost everything else in your life, the more you multitask, the worse you are at it."
—Peter Bregman

Single-tasking reduces your stress level and actually saves time. I often forget this, try to tackle way too much, and lose my mind (and my keys) in the process.

I absolutely love what Peter Bregman says about multitasking in his book, *18 Minutes*. He shares, "We don't actually multitask, we switch-task. And it's inefficient, unproductive, and sometimes even dangerous. Resist the temptation."

More inspiration:
* *18 Minutes: Find Your Focus, Master Distraction, and Get the Right Things Done* by Peter Bregman
* *The Power of Less: The Fine Art of Limiting Yourself to the Essential…in Business and in Life* by Leo Babauta

Affirmation:
I single-task whenever I can. I feel more relaxed when I choose this lifestyle.

To explore …

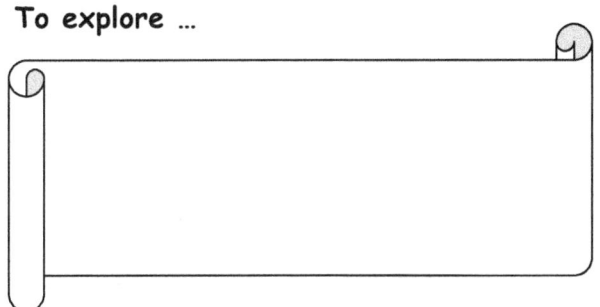

Energizing Idea 10:
Eat small meals every 3–4 hours.

*"Want to learn how to eat a lot? Here it is:
Eat a little. That way, you will be around
long enough to eat a lot."*
—Tony Robbins

Eating small meals every three hours keeps your blood sugar steady. Include a complex carbohydrate (like whole-grain bread, nuts, seeds, fruits and vegetables, or beans), protein, and water.

Eating at regular intervals keeps your metabolism burning all day long. This is the secret weapon in maintaining a healthy weight and a consistent energy level. Start with the healthiest breakfast humanly possible for an awesome day!

More inspiration:

- *Just the Rules: Tosca's Guide to Eating Right* by Tosca Reno
- *Small Changes, Big Results* by Ellie Krieger and Kelly James-Enger

Affirmation:
I nourish my body with frequent healthy meals.

To explore …

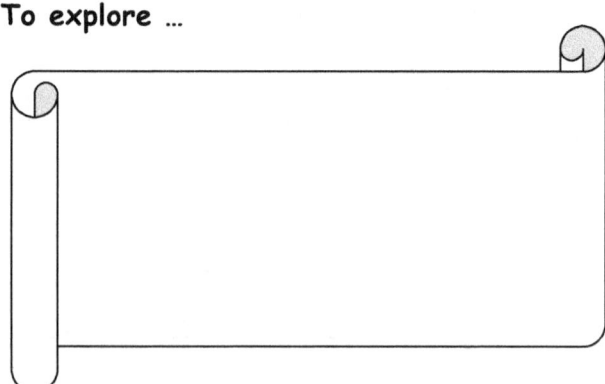

Energizing Idea 11:
Do the toughest item
on your list first.

*"The journey of a thousand miles
starts with a single step."*
—Lao Tzu

When I turned 40, I started to take amazing care of myself. (Why did I wait so long?) The first change I made was to exercise before my family woke up. At the time, I disliked exercise of any kind and getting it done early checked a big item off my list. Fifteen years later, I still exercise at 5:30 a.m., but now it's because I enjoy it immensely … who knew it would be this much fun?

What do I want to tackle first thing in the morning? How can I make it happen?

_____
_____
_____
_____
_____

More inspiration:
* *Eat That Frog: 21 Great Ways to Stop Procrastinating and Get More Done in Less Time* by Brian Tracy
* *The Success Principles: How to Get From Where You Are to Where You Want to Be* by Jack Canfield and Janet Switzer

Affirmation:
I avoid procrastinating; there's no time like the present to start!

Energizing Idea 12:
Write a heartfelt thank-you note.

"I would thank you from the bottom of my heart, but for you my heart has no bottom."
—Author Unknown

Delight in expressing your gratitude with a note. (The recipient may be alive or dead.) Enjoy the tears, the smiles, and the giggles bubbling to the surface as you share your feelings. Don't hold back. Feel the loving energy.

Consider taking a minute each day to silently thank those you hold dear. I can't think of a better use of 60 seconds. The happiest people are those who practice feeling grateful.

More inspiration:
* *Gratitude: A Way of Life* by Louise Hay and Friends
* *The Way of Happy Woman: Living the Best Year of Your Life* by Sara Avant Stover
* Your gratitude journal and loving thoughts

Affirmation:

I express my gratitude freely and lovingly. Abundance flows into my life in surprising ways every day.

"If the only prayer you said in your life was 'thank you,' that would suffice."
—Meister Eckhart

Energizing Idea 13:
Eat less meat!
Try "Meatless Mondays."

"Nothing will benefit human health and increase chances for a survival of life on Earth as much as the evolution to a vegetarian diet."
—Albert Einstein

If you are a meat eater, consider going meatless every Monday. It's a way for your body to experience some interesting healthy alternatives. Notice how you feel. (Do you have more energy? Feel lighter? Have less digestion issues? Eat fewer calories and feel more satisfied?)

Eating less meat is a great way to lower your cholesterol, reduce your risk of chronic illness, and lessen your carbon footprint.

Research shows, when we start a healthy habit on a Monday we are more likely to continue during the week.

More inspiration:

- *The Engine 2 Diet* by Rip Esselstyn
- www.MeatlessMonday.com
- *Veganist: Lose Weight, Get Healthy, Change the World* by Kathy Freston

Affirmation:

I choose healthy foods to feed my mind and body.

To explore ...

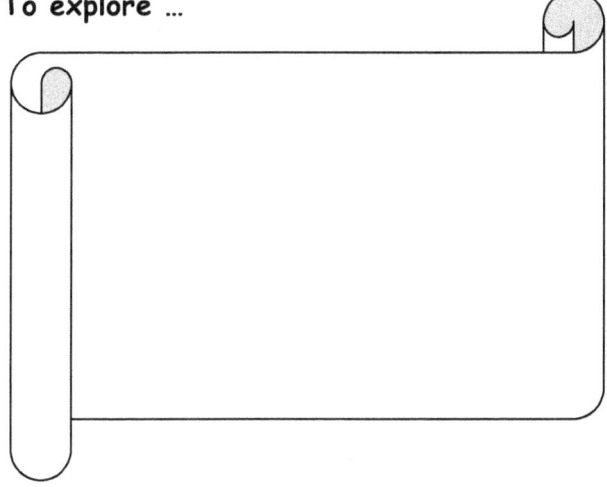

Energizing Idea 14:
Find ways to de-stress.

*"Stress is like an iceberg. We can see
one-eighth of it above,
but what about what's below?"*
—Author Unknown

Ideas for de-stressing:

* Know your limits. Be realistic about what you can accomplish in a day.
* Listen to soothing music, a friend, or both.
* Don't procrastinate … it facilitates feeling stressed!
* Exercise, meditate, practice yoga, walk, or dance.
* Read. Look at art. Take photos.
* Enjoy a relaxing bath.
* Breathe in/out slowly. Repeat.
* Don't worry about what you can't change.
* Eat healthy food. Take your vitamins. Get enough sleep.

More inspiration:

* *Relax & De-Stress* (Music for Self-Healing) Audio CD by Dr. Andrew Weil and Joshua Leeds
* *Positive Energy: 10 Extraordinary Prescriptions for Transforming Fatigue, Stress and Fear into Vibrance, Strength, and Love* by Judith Orloff

Affirmation:
I reduce my stress by …

_____

_____

Energizing Idea 15:
Hang around energetic, enthusiastic, active people.

"Whether they burst with excitement or simmer quietly, when you're in the presence of enthusiastic people, you feel happier and more excited about your life, perhaps you even feel inspired."
—Mary Marcdante

Energetic, enthusiastic, active people are less likely to develop heart disease than those who are not. Will this health benefit "rub off" on you when you enjoy their friendship? I hope so! We definitely need enthusiastic people to light up our lives!

More inspiration:
- www.MaryMarcdante.com
- *Exuberance: The Passion for Life* by Kay Redfield Jamison

Affirmation:
I delight in spending time with energetic, enthusiastic, active people.

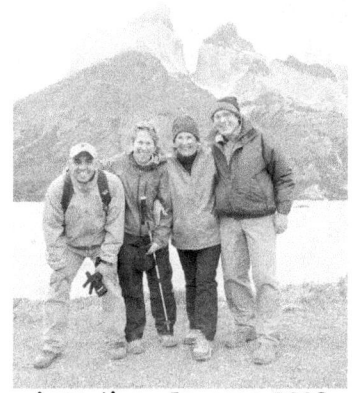

Argentina, January 2008

Energizing Idea 16:
If you are overweight,
lose weight sensibly.

*"I keep trying to lose weight ...
but it keeps finding me!"*
—Author Unknown

Research and decide on a food and exercise plan
that makes sense to you. Stick with it. Ask for help
along the journey.

Concentrate on your most important reason(s). For
example: your improved health, your increased
energy, and your overall feeling of wellness.
(This leads to more success than losing weight for
vanity's sake.)

More inspiration:

- *YOU: Losing Weight: The Owner's Manual to
  Simple and Healthy Weight Loss* by Michael
  Roizen, M.D. and Mehmet Oz, M.D.
- *Eat to Live: The Amazing Nutrient-Rich Program
  for Fast and Sustained Weight Loss* by Joel
  Fuhrman, M.D.

Affirmation:

I strive to maintain a healthy weight for my
body by ...
_____
_____

To explore ...

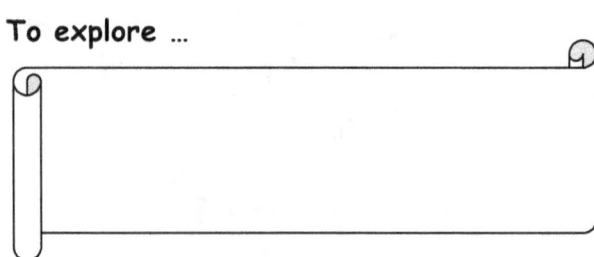

Energizing Idea 17:
For a quick pick-me-up,
eat some raw, unsalted nuts.

"I grab a handful of walnuts or almonds whenever I'm hungry. The protein and healthy fat help keep me satiated and provide me with lots of energy through the day. Best of all, recent research suggests that we don't digest all the calories in nuts, so we actually get a bit of caloric discount when we eat them."
—Mehmet Oz, M.D.

- Nuts are packed with omega-3 fats, which improve mood and brain function essential for avoiding a midday slump.
- They are one of the best sources of protein.
- Nuts are rich in fiber, phytonutrients, and antioxidants.
- Flax seeds, pumpkin seeds, and sunflower seeds are great, too!
- Use nuts as a replacement for other high saturated-fat snack foods.

More inspiration:
- www.Sunfood.com
- Your favorite markets

Affirmation:
I take special care to listen to my body and feed it what it needs to be healthy.

Energizing Idea 18:
Apply basic feng shui principles.

"When you live and work in places that feel good to you, your attitude becomes more positive and the quality of your life improves."
—Cathleen McCandless

Feng shui (pronounced fung-SHWAY) is the art of placing things in your home and office to facilitate the circulation of chi (vital energy.) The Chinese believe when your chi is circulating freely in your environment your energy level will be high. If your chi is blocked, you will feel tired.

Some simple tips:

- Add a fish tank or fish bowl with brightly colored fish to your living room or other quiet, meditative area.

- Display healthy, vibrant flowers, or plants (real or silk.)

- Avoid placing exercise equipment, computers, and work materials in your bedroom. This is your place to rest.

- Keep bedroom lighting soft (consider a dimmer switch and/or nontoxic candles.) Please keep fresh air circulating.

- Using brown and green colors in your living room promotes health and vitality.

Anything you can do to decorate in a simple uplifting way, with as little clutter as possible, will help you create a space in which you will feel healthier.

More inspiration:

- *Feng Shui That Makes Sense—Easy Ways to Create A Home That Feels as Good as It Looks* by Cathleen McCandless

- www.TheSpiritualFengShui.com (informative newsletters)

Affirmation:

I surround myself with simplicity and beauty. I love how I feel.

To explore ...

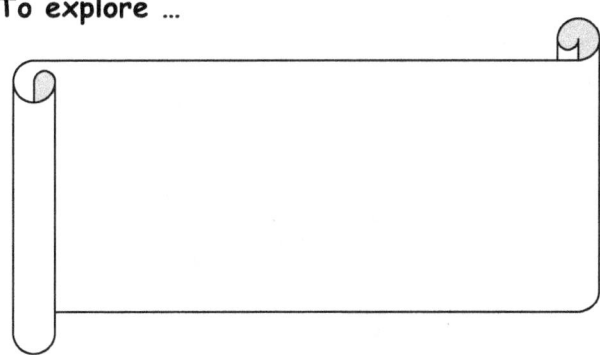

Energizing Idea 19:
Move your body!

"Find your comfort zone with exercise and work within it. Reassess your comfort zone on a regular basis, at least monthly. You will find that as you get smaller, your comfort zone will get larger."
—Amy Culver

Human bodies are designed for regular physical activity. Any kind of movement will power you up. Try a walk inside or outside for a quick pick-me-up. Keep active. (Do lunges while you are on the phone. Take the stairs instead of the elevator.) Engage in the movement activities that bring a smile to your face. You'll love the energy boost.

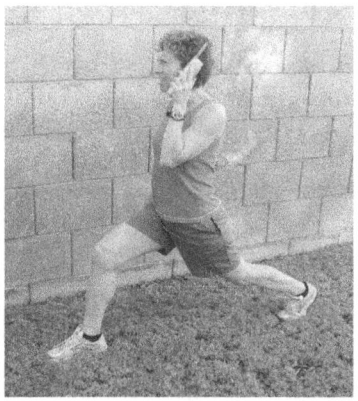

More inspiration:

- *Spark: The Revolutionary New Science of Exercise and the Brain* by John J. Ratey and Eric Hagerman
- *Mindful Movements: Ten Exercises for Well-Being* by Thich Nhat Hanh

Affirmation:

I move my body and love how being active feels.

Energizing Idea 20:
Drink a green smoothie.

"Vegetables are the food of the earth;
fruit seems more the food of the heavens."
—Sepal Felicivant

Here's a green smoothie recipe that is a real winner:

- 1 medium banana
- 1/2 cup frozen berries
- 1 cup fresh baby spinach
- 1 cup unsweetened soy milk
- 2 teaspoons raw almond butter

Blend until smooth. Enjoy!

This recipe creates a fantastic, 14-ounce, purple-colored smoothie, perfect to share with a loved one any time of day. It's so delicious ... you would never guess it's healthy.

Experiment with different ingredients and quantities. I enjoy using unsweetened frozen fruit and no ice. Avoid pesticides by purchasing organic fruits and vegetables whenever you can.

More inspiration:
- *Green Smoothie Revolution: The Radical Leap Towards Natural Health* by Victoria Boutenko
- *Rawlicious* by Peter and Beryn Daniel

Affirmation:
Drinking a green smoothie powers up my body.

Editor's note: When asked for feedback on *All-Day Energy*, I told Syd I was willing to try all the ideas except this one. She laughed and didn't pressure me, but just before publication time I tried her recipe and, you know what ... it tasted great!

Energizing Idea 21:
Accept yourself as you are.

"We are already perfect as we are:
perfectly imperfect, that is."
—Taro Gold

Many years ago, my friend Kae shared this lovely story:

> An elderly woman had two large pots, each hung on the ends of a pole, which she carried across her neck. One of the pots had a crack in it while the other pot was perfect and always delivered a full portion of water.
>
> At the end of the long walk from the stream to her house, the cracked pot arrived only half full. For a full two years this went on daily, with the woman bringing home only one-and-a-half pots of water. Of course, the perfect pot was proud of its accomplishments. But the poor cracked pot was ashamed of its own imperfection, and miserable that it could only do half of what it had been made to do.
>
> After two years of what it perceived to be a bitter failure, it spoke to the women by the stream. It said, "I am ashamed of myself, because this crack in my side causes water to leak out all the way back to your house."
>
> The old woman smiled. She replied, "Did you notice that there are flowers on your side of the path, but not on the other pot's side? That's because I have always known about your flaw, so I planted flower seeds on your side of the path, and every day while we walk back, you water them. For two years, I have been able to pick these beautiful flowers to decorate the table. Without you being just the way you are, there would not be this beauty to grace our house."

I love this story! Each of us has our own unique flaws. But it's the cracks and flaws we each have that make our lives together so very interesting and rewarding.

More inspiration:

- *Living Wabi Sabi: The True Beauty of Your Life* by Taro Gold
- *A Deep Breath of Life: Daily Inspiration for Heart-Centered Living* by Alan Cohen

Affirmation:

I love and accept myself exactly as I am, with joy and gratitude.

To explore ...

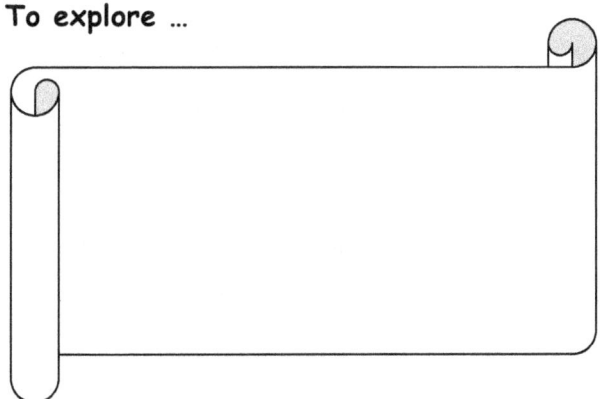

Energizing Idea 22:
Take high-quality vitamins.

"Friendship is like vitamins, we supplement
each other's minimum daily requirements."
—Author Unknown

Although I eat a very healthy array of fruits,
vegetables and other nutritious food, I am a firm
believer in taking quality supplements. Our foods,
even fresh whole foods, simply no longer have the
nutrition we need to stay healthy. For example, in a
recent study, scientists found you need to eat 26
peaches to get the same levels of Vitamin A from
only one peach in 1951. Did you have your 26
peaches today?

Our bodies are designed to gain nutrients from
plant-based foods. Ninety-five percent of the
nutritional supplement market in America uses
synthetic (made in a chemical laboratory) or
inorganic ingredients we cannot absorb. These
include coal tar and petroleum byproducts, and
minerals from rocks. I have found two science-
based nutritional companies with products
containing plant-based vitamins and minerals:
Mannatech and Vemma.

I began taking Mannatech "Optimal Support
Packets" about 10 years ago. It's a simple way to
get my daily minerals, vitamins, antioxidants, and
nutrients to support my endocrine, immune,
nervous, and cardiovascular system health.
Mannatech supplement packets have five easy-to-
swallow pills providing glyconutrients missing from
our diet.

When I travel, I enjoy drinking immune-boosting Vemma Mangosteen Plus. The two-ounce bottles are a convenient source of vitamins, minerals, and energy. Vemma has no artificial sweeteners, colors, or flavors. It's free of gluten and preservatives. Vemma is a nice addition to my daily Mannatech supplements.

More inspiration:

- www.Vemma.com
- www.MannatechScience.org
- Best product prices: www.LowestCostStore.com

Affirmation:

Vitamins and minerals help every cell in my body function properly. I feel incredible!

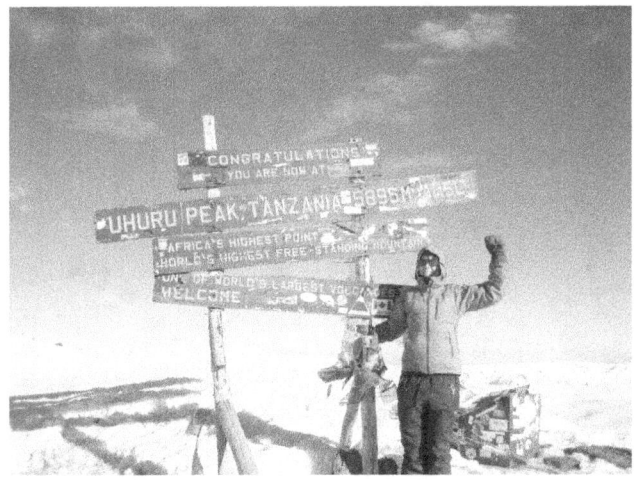

**Here's my Mt. Kilimanjaro summit photo ...
happy, strong, and vibrant at age 50!
February 2007**

Energizing Idea 23:
Stroll through a farmers' market.

"There must be more to life than increasing its speed."
—Mahatma Gandhi

What could be better than all the sights, smells, and sounds of a farmers' market? It's a great way to meet those amazing people who grow organic fruits and vegetables right in your own backyard. Often there are artisans selling jewelry, paintings, and other items. Stroll through. Sample fabulous foods. Shake hands. Smile. Be grateful. Purchase joyfully. There are more than 7,000 farmers' markets in America.

Where are the closest farmers' markets to my home or office? When are they open?

_____
_____
_____

More inspiration:
* www.LocalHarvest.org (to find markets near you)
* *The Harvest Eating Cookbook* by Keith Snow

Affirmation:
How delightful it is to eat locally grown healthy food and support my local merchants!

Energizing Idea 24:
Treat yourself to a face mask.

"Nature gives you the face you have at 20;
it is up to you to merit
the face you have at 50."
—Coco Chanel

Facial masks have been used since ancient times. They rejuvenate your skin and help you feel pampered. I love to treat myself to a face mask on Sunday evening ... it's such a pleasant way to start the week.

You can purchase an inexpensive mask at your local store or online. I like to use them but I also enjoy making a homemade face mask.

A nice recipe is 1 egg white and 1 tablespoon of plain yogurt. For a grittier mask, combine 2 teaspoons of instant oatmeal with a teaspoon of baking soda ... add water to make a paste. The second mask is messier but it feels great!

Experiment, explore, and most importantly have fun!

Affirmation:
I make time to take care of my face.

Energizing Idea 25:
Take a brisk walk.

*"It is impossible to walk rapidly
and be unhappy."*
—Mother Teresa

I love to walk. I encourage everyone I meet to give it a try.

Ideas for fitting a walk into your day:
- Exit your bus a stop earlier and walk the rest of the way.
- Keep walking shoes and sneakers in your car ready for action.
- Lay out your clothes the night before and grab a walk before your family wakes up.
- Walk before (or after) lunch or dinner with a loved one, a pet, or both.
- Sign up for a 5K or 10K walk with a buddy; train together at least once a week.

Interesting fact:
You'll feel revved up for **two hours** after taking just a 10-minute walk!

More inspiration:
- www.Walking.About.com
- *The Complete Guide to Walking for Health, Weight Loss, and Fitness* by Mark Fenton

Affirmation:
I walk to connect with myself, nature, and ...

_____

_____

_____

Energizing Idea 26:
Take a nap.

*"No day is so bad
it can't be fixed with a nap."*
—Carrie P. Snow

Brain efficiency naturally drops after lunch. A short nap recharges your "battery" and adds loads of extra mental oomph for the remainder of your day.

Even naps as short as 10 minutes have been shown to reduce fatigue and improve concentration. (Imagine what 20–30 minutes will do!)

A large number of people all over the world benefit from an afternoon "siesta." History is full of famous nappers, including these creative minds:

- Thomas Edison
- Winston Churchill
- John F. Kennedy
- Napoleon Bonaparte
- Albert Einstein
- Leonardo Da Vinci

My favorite days are when I have time for a 15-minute pre-lunch brisk walk, a healthy lunch and then a nap. What a mood booster and energy-enhancing trio!

More inspiration:
- www.WikiHow.com/nap
- *Take a Nap! Change Your Life.* by Sara Mednick Ph.D. and Mark Ehrman

Affirmation:
Naps refresh me.

Energizing Idea 27:
Get a bodywork treatment: a massage, acupuncture, or chiropractic adjustment.

"Tension is who you think you should be. Relaxation is who you are."
—Chinese Proverb

I invest in my health by getting a massage from Reggie every four weeks. He "tenderizes" my muscles in a way that is different from yoga, pilates, and stretching. It's an excellent way to relax overused muscles. Bodywork will:

- Help eliminate harmful toxins
- Boost your immune system

Treat your body well and watch your energy soar and pains fly away!

More inspiration:
- www.MassageTherapy.com
- www.Acupuncture.com
- www.Chiropractic.org

Affirmation:
I see and feel the benefits of bodywork.

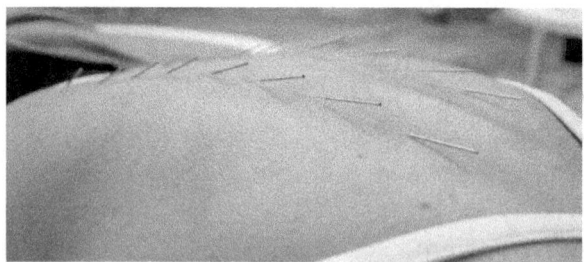

Original color photo by
Victoria Garcia (www.ggvic.com).
Acupuncture needles in her mom's back.

Energizing Idea 28:
Follow your passion.

"Don't ask what the world needs. Ask what makes you come alive, and go do it. Because what the world needs is people who come alive."
—Howard Thurman

When you follow your passion you are:

- More motivated and alive
- Generally happier
- Able to build on what you already know
- A better idea-generator

What makes me come alive …

_____

_____

_____

_____

_____

More inspiration:

- *What's Next? Follow your Passion and Find Your Dream Job* by Kerry Hannon
- www.FYBmag.com

Affirmation:

I know that when I follow my passion all is right with the world.

Energizing Idea 29:
Read an informative magazine online, at the library, or by subscription.

"Reading is a means of thinking with another person's mind; it forces you to stretch your own."
—Charles Scribner, Jr.

I enjoy my magazine subscriptions. It's a great way for me to keep up with world news, new health trends, and what's happening in the yoga community. If you have interests you want to learn more about, consider reading a magazine.

I like to dog-ear corners of articles, tab the magazine with post-it notes, and write on the cover. Some magazines get saved, others get separated. I donate a lot of my "unmarked" magazines to my public library for them to resell.

Resources for new and gently used magazines:
- Your local public library
- Your local bookstore or recycled goods store.

Magazines I enjoy ...

_____
_____
_____

I'd like to find magazines on these topics ...

_____
_____
_____

Affirmation:
Reading a magazine energizes my brain with nuggets of information.

Energizing Idea 30:
Carry your mini-meals with you.

"He who fails to plan is planning to fail."
—Winston Churchill

Pack your day's meals in a portable insulated food bag. You'll have the strength to avoid the vending machines. And you will be able to use the extra cash to spend on smaller-sized clothing.

I usually pack two pieces of fresh fruit, a sandwich on sprouted bread (or a salad), a handful of nuts, a green smoothie, hummus and fresh veggies. Add a cloth napkin, utensils, and water. You'll eat like royalty all day long.

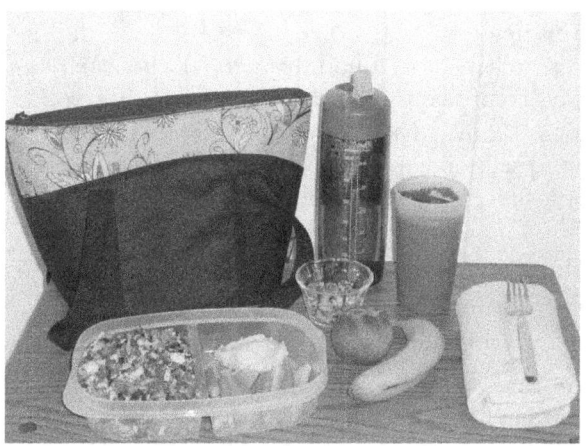

More inspiration:
- *Just The Rules!* by Tosca Reno
- *The Abs Diet Eat Right Every Time Guide* by David Zinczenko

Affirmation:
I take the time to plan what I'm going to eat … I'm worth it!

Energizing Idea 31:
Sing in your car.
(In the shower, too!)

"When in doubt, sing loud."
—Robert Merrill

There would be a lot less road rage if people would sing while they drive. Who cares if you can carry a tune? No one is listening.

Singing in the car makes me smile. I'm a low-tech person ... I use the radio or CDs for my car music. I'm always surprised when a favorite song comes on. I'll sing it proudly ... even if I don't know the words!

Amazing fact:
Researchers have found that people who listen to their favorite music for an hour every other week for a few months can lower their blood pressure by up to six points ... equal to going on a low-salt diet or losing 10 pounds. Wow!

More inspiration:

- Music websites: www.iTunes.com, www.Pandora.com, www.Rhapsody.com, www.Spotify.com
- Your radio, favorite CDs, and other high-tech players!

Affirmation:
Singing is a lot of fun. It always makes me smile.

Energizing Idea 32:
Eat a healthy breakfast at home.

"You have solemn obligation to take care of
yourself because you never know
when the world will need you."
—Rabbi Hillel

People who eat a healthy breakfast are more
energetic than those who don't. Sharpen your
memory and mental clarity all day long with that
special first meal of the day!

Mornings can be hectic. Consider preparing for
breakfast the night before by defrosting a small
portion of assorted (unsweetened) frozen fruit in
your refrigerator. (Last night, I took a few
moments to combine pineapple, blueberries,
raspberries, and peaches.) In the morning, you have
a ready-to-go topping for plain yogurt or oatmeal.

I love eating "real" oatmeal for breakfast. Start with
rolled oats … not anything quick or instant. Buy
100 percent whole-grain oats, gluten free, wheat
free and dairy free. Some brands have more fiber
than steel-cut oats (e.g. Trader Joe's). Prepare as
directed, or try my delicious time-saving method:
Combine 1/2 cup oats, 1 cup unsweetened almond
milk (any type of milk works), a little cinnamon,
and vanilla in a covered medium-sized glass bowl,
refrigerate overnight. Microwave to warm if desired.

Start your day with the winning combination of a
lean protein and a complex carbohydrate. If you are
not a "breakfast person," try a smoothie, a salad, a
sandwich … whatever works for you.

Affirmation:
I start my day off right with a healthy breakfast and
I feel vibrant all day long.

Energizing Idea 33:
Lift weights 2-3 times per week.

"Strength training will help you avoid injury and keep your metabolism running in high gear by building muscle."
—Bob Greene

When I turned 45, I decided to lift weights to ensure I did not lose bone density as I aged. After a couple of months, I realized **many** things got "lifted" … my energy, my strength, and my mood. I also noticed my posture improved. My body was more toned … shapelier. (I finally had the confidence to wear a sleeveless top.) I experienced first-hand that more muscle mass means more calories burned!

Give it a try at home or in your local fitness center. If you are a beginner, be sure to ask for help developing a 20–30 minute plan. Learn how to maintain proper alignment for maximum efficiency and safety. Please don't wait until you reach the age of 45 to begin.

Fun tip:
Add 30–60 seconds of aerobic exercise between weight lifting sets to burn 30 percent more calories.

More inspiration:
* www.LiveStrong.com
* Your local fitness center
* *The New Rules of Lifting* by Lou Schuler and Alwyn Cosgrove

The days I lift weights are …

_____

_____

_____

If I need help with strength training, I can ask …

_____

_____

_____

Other thoughts, resources, and things to investigate …

_____

_____

_____

Affirmation:

I keep my body lean and strong by lifting weights.

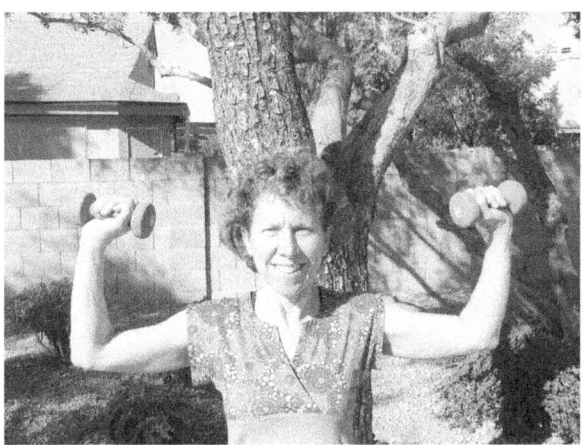

Energizing Idea 34:
Visualize your success.

"Visualize this thing that you want, see it, feel it, believe in it. Make it your mental blueprint, and begin to build."
—Robert Collier

Visualization is a successful technique used by people in all walks of life. Decide what you really want and put your imagination to work. You can use visualization to replace old habits or to acquire new ones. It's useful in achieving goals, finding employment, accomplishing your dreams, and so much more.

Visualize where you would like to be in six months, a year, two years, and five years. Give yourself the gift of patience and calmness. For best results, visualize often.

More inspiration:
- *Want it, See It, Get It! Visualize Your Way to Success* by Gini Graham Scott
- *Think and Grow Rich* by Napoleon Hill

Affirmation:
I visualize what I want and the Universe starts paving the path for me to get there.

To explore ...

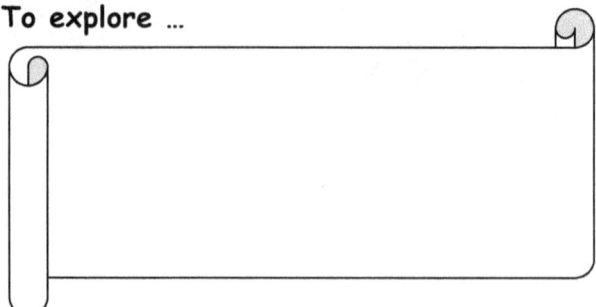

Energizing Idea 35:
Journal your joy, your gratitude, your dreams, and your successes.

"Even after all this time, the Sun never says to the Earth, 'You owe me.' Look at what happens with a love like that; it lights the whole sky."
—Hafiz

Keeping a gratitude journal increases your happiness level. It will change how you view the miracles that occur each day in your life.

Consider journal writing daily or several times a week. I really enjoy the gratitude journal we write in at home together. We started it November 2011. It's a beautiful collection of our appreciation for day-to-day events, people, and so much more.

More inspiration:
- *Make Miracles in Forty Days* by Melody Beattie
- *Living in Gratitude* by Angeles Arrien
- *Gratitude: The Essential Practice for Happiness & Fulfillment* by Angeles Arrien (audio CD)

Affirmation:
I express my joy and gratitude freely.

02/21/12   Journal entr
    I am grateful for how you honor my
silly requests - like dancing in the kitchen
at 9am, going for a mid-day walk, or
kissing as the Vitamix blends our smoothies.
You bring sunshine to my day! XO

Energizing Idea 36:
Decide on your menu selection before you arrive at a restaurant.

"We can make a commitment to promote vegetables, fruit, and whole grains on every part of every menu. We can make portion sizes smaller and emphasize quality over quantity. And we can help create a culture—imagine this—where our kids ask for healthy options instead of resisting them."
—Michelle Obama

It's so easy to choose the wrong meal or to eat too much when we go to a restaurant. The temptation to eat everything on our plate and split huge desserts with our friends is just too strong. When we decide ahead of time *exactly* what we are ordering, and what portion goes right in the take-home box, we're setting ourselves up for a happy, confident experience. No regrets during or after the meal. No need for will power ... it's all planned ahead of time.

Most restaurants have their menu online. Some have the nutritional value of each dish as well. Anything on the menu can be added or deleted from your selection. Ask politely. You are the guest.

Unusual tip to try:
When you are at home looking at the menu, jot down exactly what you plan to order on an index card. Be specific. Here are my notes for lunch at the Phoenix Art Museum café:

"Farmers' Market Salad" with balsamic dressing on the side (tahini or hummus instead of dressing, if available). No bread & butter. (Substitute: wheat flaxseed crackers.) Water with lemon.

Pure joy!

Affirmation:
I respect that my body needs just the right fuel to be its healthiest.

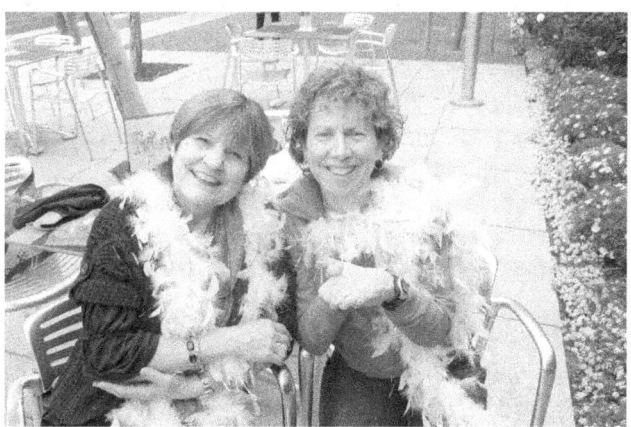

Wild Sandra and I at the
Phoenix Art Museum café.

Energizing Idea 37:
Watch your sugar and caffeine intake.

*"Good communication is just as
stimulating as black coffee,
and just as hard to sleep after."*
—Anne Morrow Lindbergh

Sugary desserts are the enemy of healthy eating, but sugar has a way of entering our body many other ways. Become an avid label reader. Be careful of processed peanut butter, flavored yogurts, cereals, granolas, energy bars, canned soups, canned fruit, and sauces. Avoid corn syrup, alcohol, and other refined sugars.

Beverages and foods containing caffeine are quick to raise your energy levels but can interrupt your sleep cycle, causing you to gravitate toward unhealthy snacks and caffeine the next day to battle yesterday's residual fatigue. Consider weaning yourself off caffeine.

Affirmation:
I limit my sugar and caffeine intake to maximize my all-day energy.

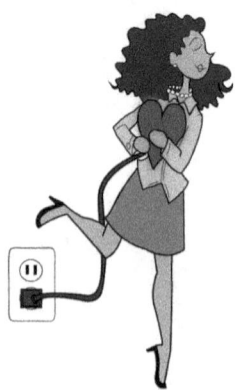

Energizing Idea 38:
Jot down today's "rough plan" and keep it in view.

"Setting a goal is not the main thing. It is deciding how you will go about achieving it and staying with the plan."
—Tom Landry

As our day goes on, we often get distracted and pulled away from the amazing plan we drafted at 6 a.m. Some changes are lovely. Others take us away from the important things we'd like to accomplish.

More inspiration:
- Your hi-tech or low-tech planner
- *What Winners Do to Win!* by Nicki Joy

Affirmation:
I keep my daily plan in plain view to help me stay focused.

To explore ...

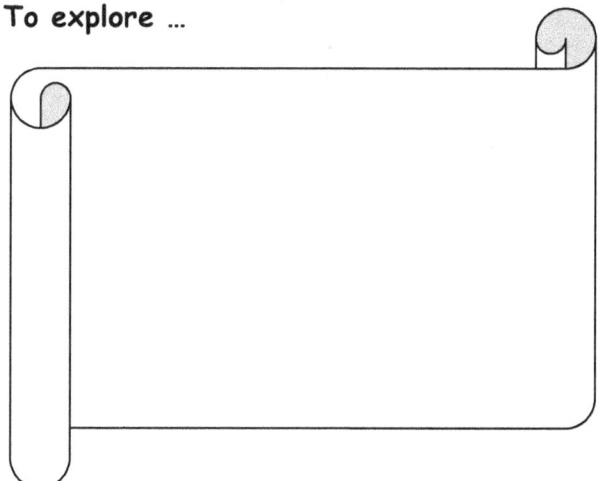

Energizing Idea 39:
Do something you enjoy.

"Just don't give up trying to do what you really want to do. Where there is love and inspiration, you can't go wrong."
—Ella Fitzgerald

Doing something you enjoy energizes your day. For me, it's being outdoors! What is it for you? What brings you joy? What makes you smile?

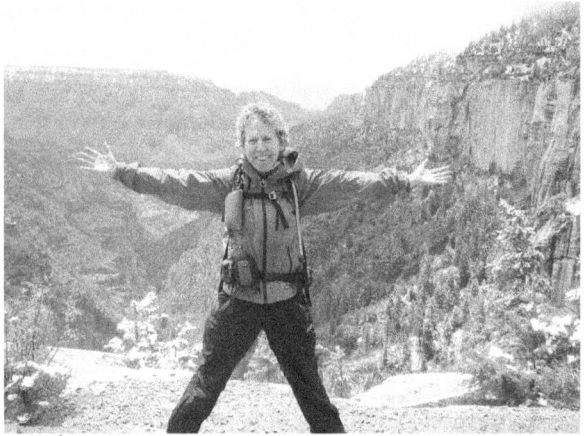

North Rim of Grand Canyon National Park, AZ, May 2011

More inspiration:
- Your favorite group of people
- Your favorite books or magazines
- Your favorite websites, places, etc.

Affirmation:
I love doing …

_____

_____

I make time for it because it's important to me … and it is fun!

Energizing Idea 40:
Split a healthy restaurant meal with a friend.

"Let your wallet stay fat, not your waist."
—Amy Culver

Restaurant portions and prices are usually "too big." And I'd like to keep this body from getting too large. So ... I share a lunch or dinner item with one or two friends. The conversation is lively and the meal is a perfect size. We leave the restaurant satisfied, but not feeling like we can't lift our bodies up from the table because we're too stuffed. No doggie bag to refrigerate. No huge bill.

More inspiration:
* www.HappyCow.net (a free fabulous online guide for choosing healthy restaurants and supermarkets)
* *Ultrametabolism* by Mark Hyman, M.D.

Affirmation:
I love to eat with friends! I feel so healthy sharing and eating smaller meals.

To explore ...

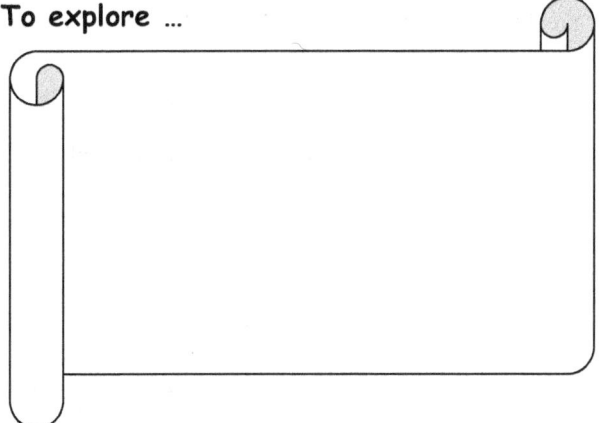

Energizing Idea 41:
Find peace in simplicity.

*"Simplicity is not the opposite of wealth.
It is the door to the riches you
already own."*
—Alan Cohen

Linda Breen Pierce has a delightful "prescription for a simple life." Her list includes: journaling, living in a different place for several months, choosing only material things you absolutely love, spending time in nature, shortening your commute to work, connecting with a sense of spirit, and practicing saying no. She's a very wise woman!

My thoughts on simplicity:

_____
_____
_____
_____
_____
_____

More inspiration:
* *Simple Abundance* by Sarah Breathnach
* *Choosing Simplicity: Real People Finding Peace and Fulfillment in a Complex World* by Linda Breen Pierce

Affirmation:
I am enjoying every step on the road to simplicity.

Energizing Idea 42:
Boost your immune system.

"What we eat has everything to do with our health and, unfortunately, too many of us are living with a severely depleted immune system."
—Joel Fuhrman, M.D.

Follow these sensible living guidelines:

- Don't smoke.
- Eat plenty of servings of fruits and vegetables.
- Exercise a minimum of three times a week. Keep active.
- Maintain a healthy weight.
- Control your blood pressure.
- If you drink alcohol, drink only in moderation.
- Get adequate sleep.
- Take steps to avoid infection.
- Get regular medical screening tests.

No one specific food item provides all the minerals and vitamins needed for a strong immune system. Each "top immunity-boosting foods" list varies slightly, but the best foods include: yogurt, oats, barley, garlic, leafy vegetables, omega-3 enriched foods, green tea, sweet potatoes, and mushrooms.

More inspiration:
- *Super Immunity* by Joel Fuhrman, M.D.
- *Super Immunity Foods* by Frances Sheridan Goulart

Affirmation:
I strengthen my immune system by eating healthy foods and exercising regularly.

Energizing Idea 43:
Think positively.

"Keep your thoughts positive, because your thoughts become your words. Keep your words positive, because your words become your behavior. Keep your behavior positive, because your behavior becomes your habits. Keep your habits positive, because your habits become your values. Keep your values positive, because your values become your destiny."
—Mahatma Gandhi

Start your day with positive thoughts. Perhaps you have a favorite morning mantra …

_____

_____

_____

I've kept this paragraph on the importance of having a positive attitude in my wallet for many years:

> "I believe the single most significant decision I can make on a day-to-day basis is my choice of attitude. It is more important than my past, my education, my bankroll, my successes or failures, fame or pain, what other people think of me or say about me, my circumstances, or my position. Attitude keeps me going or cripples my progress. It alone fuels my fire or assaults my hope. When my attitude is right, there is no barrier too high, no valley too deep, no dream too extreme, and no challenge too great for me."
> —Charles R. Swindoll

More inspiration:

- *The Power of Positive Thinking* by Norman Vincent Peale
- *Everyday Positive Thinking* by Louise L Hay and Friends
- *The Power of Optimism* by Andy Dzurinko

Affirmation:

I look forward to sharing my positivity with the world around me.

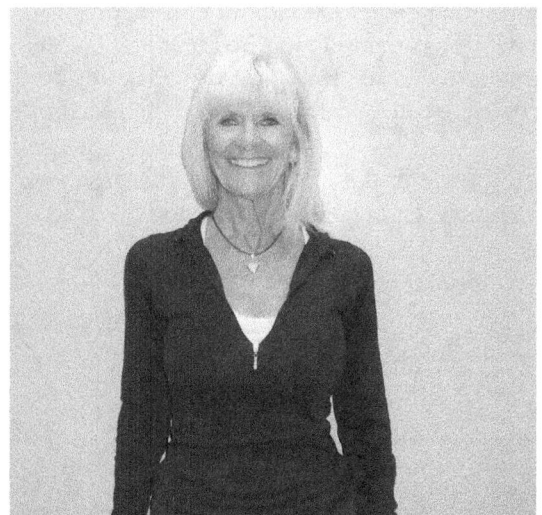

Patty, the most positive person I know!

The most positive people in my life …

_____
_____
_____
_____
_____

Energizing Idea 44:
Brainstorm.

"Nothing is more dangerous than an idea when it's the only one you've got."
—Emile-Auguste Chartier
(better known simply as Alain)

Brainstorming is the process of generating ideas without judgment or criticism. The process works well when individuals start the process alone and then brainstorm as a group. It's important to list any idea that comes up without considering whether it has merit. Don't be afraid to combine or extend ideas. Relax. Enjoy the process. Music and drawing are often useful. Be patient and kind.

I often use mind maps and graphic organizers to sort my brainstorming ideas.

For example:

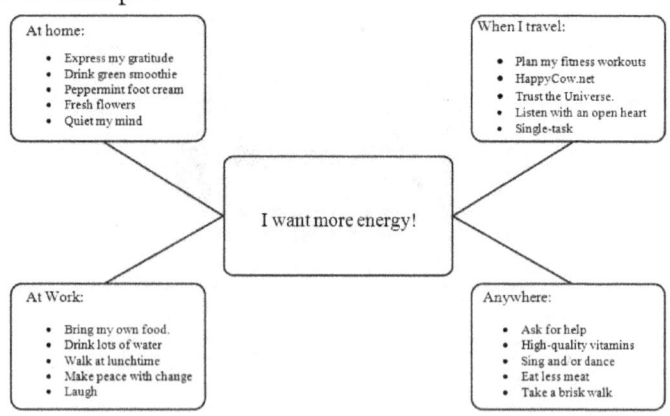

At home:
- Express my gratitude
- Drink green smoothie
- Peppermint foot cream
- Fresh flowers
- Quiet my mind

When I travel:
- Plan my fitness workouts
- HappyCow.net
- Trust the Universe.
- Listen with an open heart
- Single-task

I want more energy!

At Work:
- Bring my own food.
- Drink lots of water
- Walk at lunchtime
- Make peace with change
- Laugh

Anywhere:
- Ask for help
- High-quality vitamins
- Sing and or dance
- Eat less meat
- Take a brisk walk

Michael Bungay Stanier believes, "Too often when faced with a challenge, we seize the first idea that comes along and rush into action." I agree we need to consider more possibilities. Consider all your options ... you'll feel more energetic!

My ideas ...

_____
_____
_____

Possible action steps ...

_____
_____
_____

I'd like to brainstorm with ...

_____
_____
_____

More inspiration:
* *Do More Great Work* by Michael Bungay Stanier
* *Live More, Want Less* by Mary Carlomagno
* *Creative Whack Pack* by Roger VonOech (an illustrated card deck of 64 creative thinking strategies)

Affirmation:
I feel energetic when I use my creativity to generate new ideas!

Energizing Idea 45:
Eat a banana.

"Never interrupt me when I'm eating a banana."
—Ryan Stiles

If I had to name my favorite food, I would choose a banana. It's my "go-to" food for energy before a workout or to prevent a midday slump. I add a banana to peanut butter sandwiches, cereal, and smoothies. They are packed with dietary fiber, Vitamin C, potassium, magnesium, Vitamin B6, and are like adding dessert to every meal!

Affirmation:
What a treat to enjoy a banana instead of an unhealthy option I could have chosen!

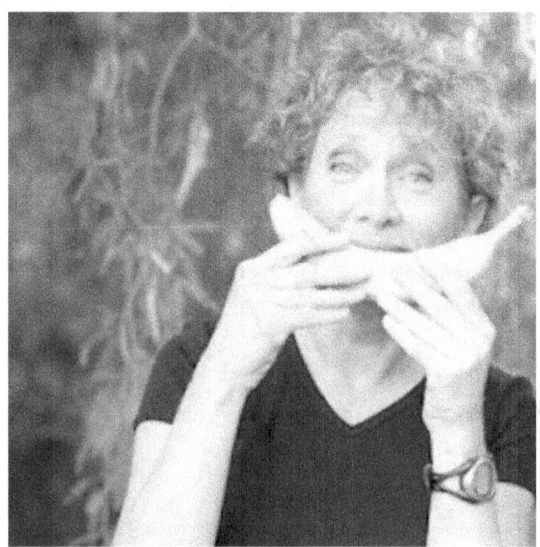

Energizing Idea 46:
Quiet your mind.

"Sit quietly, doing nothing, spring comes,
and the grass grows by itself."
—Zen saying

Try to find a small amount of time each day to
quiet your mind. It's not easy to do. Thoughts start
popping in to distract us.

If you can get past the internal clutter, you can
reach inner clarity and wisdom. The peaceful
recharge one receives from sitting quietly
is precious.

More inspiration:
* *How to Quiet Your Mind: Relax and Silence the
  Voice of Your Mind Today to Reduce Stress and
  Achieve Inner Peace Using Meditation!—
  A Beginner's Guide* by Marc Allen
* *Quiet Mind: A Beginner's Guide to Meditation*
  (book and CD set), compiled and edited by
  Susan Piver

Affirmation:
Quieting my mind is an essential practice …
it's a gift I give to myself.

To explore …

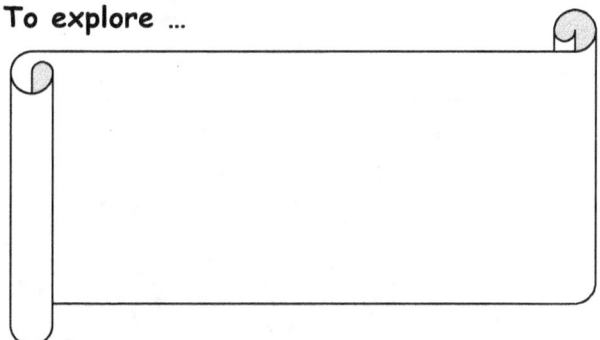

Energizing Idea 47:
Travel light.

*"When preparing to travel, lay out all your
clothes and your money. Take half the clothes
and twice the money."*
—Susan Heller

Learn to lighten your load. This is great advice for
travel, and the other important areas of your life.
Traveling light usually results in an enjoyable,
productive, and less-stressful experience.

Less stuff means greater flexibility in getting
around on public transportation, in the airport, and
at your hotel. Consider avoiding checked baggage
fees by traveling with a carry-on bag and one other
personal item. Having fewer items to keep track of
is a lovely way to relax and conserve your energy.

More inspiration:
* www.OneBag.com
* *Smart Packing for Today's Traveler*
  by Susan Foster

Affirmation:
I give myself permission to lighten my load and
experience the freedom this brings me.

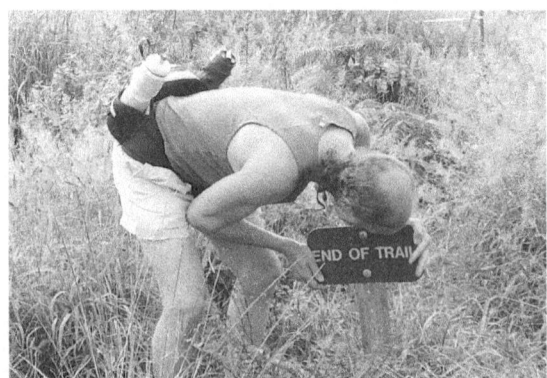

Energizing Idea 48:
Look for opportunity in every crisis.

"When written in Chinese, the word 'crisis' is composed of two characters. One represents danger and the other represents opportunity."
—John F. Kennedy

As we journey through our lives we are faced with problems and struggles. Crises encourage us to recreate ourselves, learn, and grow. These life changes help us to become our best selves.

Try to smile and recalculate. It's easier than kicking and screaming.

More inspiration:
* Your journal … write and explore
* Your friends and family

Affirmation:
I turn every experience into an opportunity.

To explore …

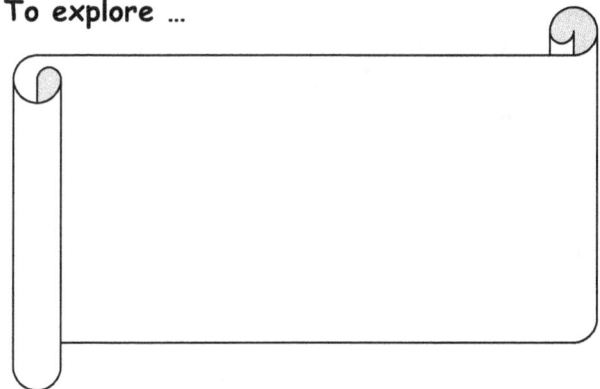

Energizing Idea 49:
Listen with an open heart.

"Our heads are round so our thoughts
can change direction."
—Francis Picabla

It's 4:15 a.m. My house is very calm and quiet. I am loving this yummy thinking-listening-writing time.

I think listening is underrated. When we truly listen to ourselves, and others, with a loving heart and an open mind, wondrous things happen! We learn. We grow. We feel. We are empowered.

L.I.S.T.E.N. Hmm, maybe it's an acronym for **Let In Sounds That Energize Naturally**.

More inspiration:
* www.JamesCPetersen.com/
  Listening_Techniques.htm
* www.DrNadig.com/listening.htm

Affirmation:
I am so grateful to have a beautiful heart and two amazing ears to truly listen to the wisdom surrounding me.

To explore ...

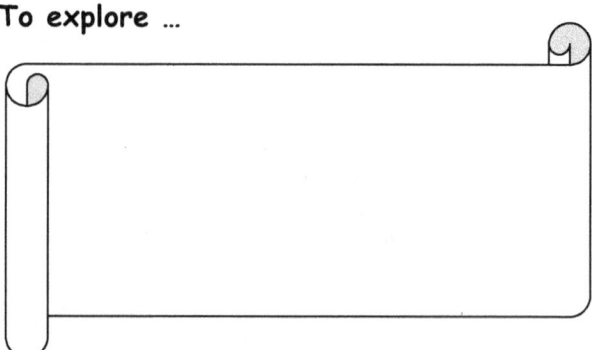

Energizing Idea 50:
Barter or hire.

"There are three ways to get something done: do it yourself, hire someone, or forbid your kids to do it."
—Monta Crane

I have a lovely bartering agreement with my friend Renee. She makes my curly hair look its best and I help her achieve her fitness goals. I'm so glad she suggested we do this!

Every two weeks, Joyful Janet (www.ChefJanetLee.com) delivers the best, unsweetened granola on the planet to our home. We happily trade her protein bars, computer services, or cash.

There are tasks that come up now and then that just aren't any fun. If you can barter or pay someone to do a dreaded job, it may just make your day delightful. (If not, just get it over with as painlessly as possible.)

More inspiration:
- www.CraigsList.org
- Your local newspaper

Affirmation:
I cheerfully barter or hire whenever possible.

Energizing Idea 51:
Look at delightful photos.

"You don't take a photograph, you make it."
—Ansel Adams

What a joy it is to sit down alone or with a dear one to look at old photos together! Our home is full of sweet photos … on the walls, on our mantel, on the computer, and in photo albums. It brings back memories, creates laughter, and adds a bounce to my step whenever I make time to gaze into a special photograph.

More inspiration:
* To learn more about photography, consider taking a class at your local community college or parks/recreation center.
* Ask your family to share photo albums with you.

Affirmation:
I enrich my life with photos—"making" them, enjoying them, and sharing them.

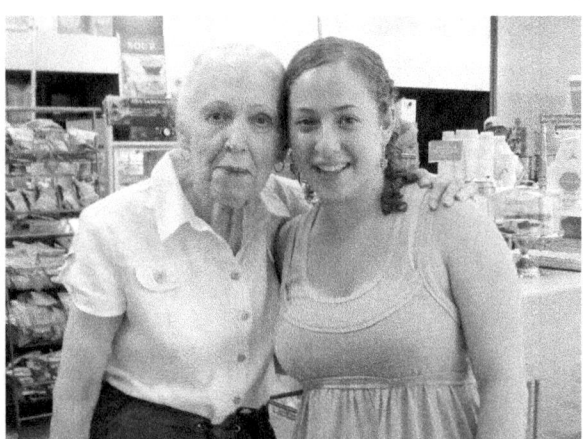

Fabulous Florence and Awesome Hillary

Energizing Idea 52:
Focus on the solution
more than the problem.

*"That the birds fly overhead, this you cannot
stop. That they build a nest in your hair,
this you can prevent."*
—Chinese Proverb

Problems stress us. Solutions energize us.

The only thing we can count on is that changes and
confusion are bound to happen in our life. Don't
let them zap your energy.

More inspiration:
* *There's a Spiritual Solution to Every Problem* by
  Wayne W. Dyer
* *Loving What Is: Four Questions That Can Change
  Your Life* by Byron Katie and Stephen Mitchell

Affirmation:
I choose to enjoy the journey and know I will solve
any problems that come up along the way.

To explore ...

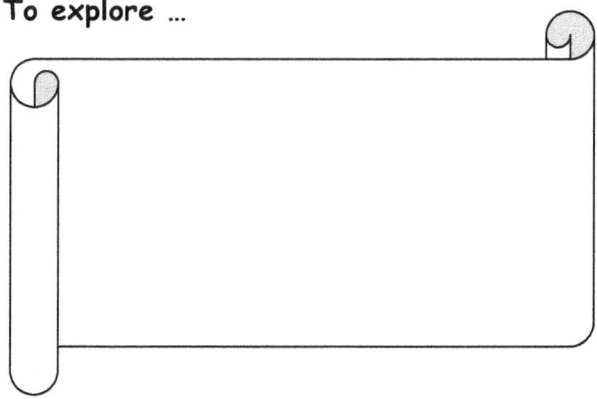

Energizing Idea 53:
Trust the Universe. Worry less.

*"I'm an old man who has known a
great many problems, most of which
never happened."*
—Mark Twain

Anxiety and mental stress deplete our physical
energy. The most common areas we worry about
are job security, the wellbeing of our children,
threat of disaster, family health, money, and
relationships.

When we plan ahead, work hard and try to be
proactive, we reduce our need to worry. So try to
journal, talk to those you trust and, most
importantly, relax when you know you've done
everything you can.

More inspiration:
- *How to Stop Worrying and Start Living*
  by Dale Carnegie
- *The Worry Solution: Using Breakthrough Brain
  Science to Turn Stress and Anxiety into Confidence
  and Happiness* by Martin Rossman, M.D.

Affirmation:
I trust the Universe.

To explore ...

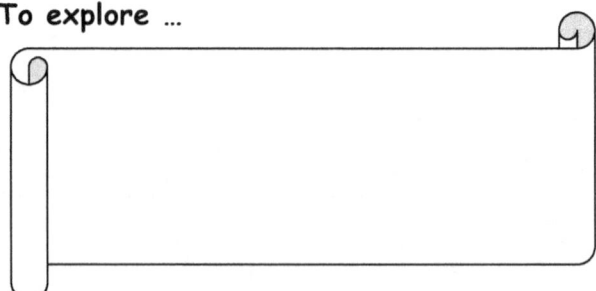

Energizing Idea 54:
Try some quinoa.

"Quinoa is a true wonder food. It has about twice the protein of regular cereal grains, fewer carbohydrates, and even a dose of healthy fats."
—Daniel Fairbanks, Ph.D.

Quinoa (pronounced KEEN-wah) is an awesome gluten-free seed that is actually a complete protein. (This means it has all nine essential amino acids.) It tastes a bit nutty, fluffs up like rice and has a slight bit of crunch. It's rich in minerals. Enjoy as a breakfast cereal, a side dish, and in your salad.

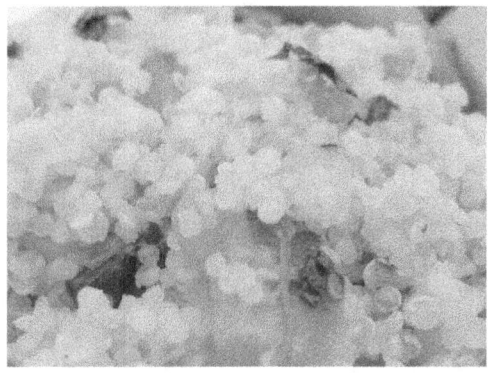

More inspiration:
- *Quinoa 101* video at www.CleanAndDelicious.com
- www.CookingQuinoa.net

Affirmation:
I love to experiment with new healthy foods. I'd like to try ...

_____

_____

_____

Energizing Idea 55:
Laugh.

Laughing is a mood booster and energizer.

Other benefits of laughter:
- Reduces blood pressure and heart rate
- Helps the body fight infection
- Releases endorphins which provide natural pain relief
- Changes your perspective
- Makes you feel good

More inspiration:
- *LOL: Laugh Out Loud—Feel Good and Live Longer* by Andy Dzurinko and James Harris
- www.LaughterYoga.org
- Joke books, funny stories, getting together with friends

Affirmation:
A day with laughter is a day well spent.

How can I add more laugher to my life and to the lives of my family and friends?

_____
_____
_____
_____
_____

Energizing Idea 56:
Get a complimentary makeup lesson.

Enjoy the experience of your makeup lesson. Take home the makeup artist's notes, including product names and colors. After waiting 48 hours, consider purchasing your favorite products. Do not feel pressured to purchase anything … today or any other day.

More inspiration:

- *Bobbi Brown Makeup Manual: For Everyone from Beginner to Pro* by Bobbi Brown

- www.Covergirl.com/Makeup-Tips

Affirmation:

I am beautiful with or without makeup.

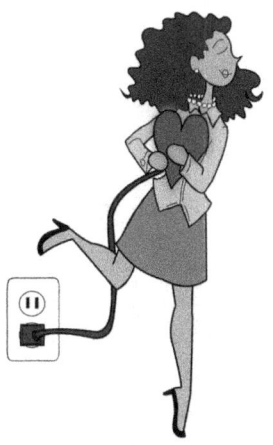

Energizing Idea 57:
Develop unflappable self-esteem.

*"No one can make you feel inferior
without your consent."*
—Eleanor Roosevelt

A healthy self-esteem is an essential ingredient for living a happy life. How we feel about ourselves affects each of our relationships and achievements.

Years ago, airport security asked passengers, "Are you carrying anything given to you by a stranger?" I think it's an important question for us to ask ourselves. Are you "carrying" any negative opinions or judgments you have picked up along the way from strangers, teachers, friends, or family members? If so, it may be time to once-and-for-all lose any dangerous "baggage."

More inspiration:
- *You Can Heal Your Life* by Louise Hay
- *The Self-Esteem Companion* by Patrick Fanning, Carole Honeychurch, Matthew McKay, Ph.D. and Catharine Sutker

Affirmation:
I am intelligent, courageous, and beautiful.

To explore …

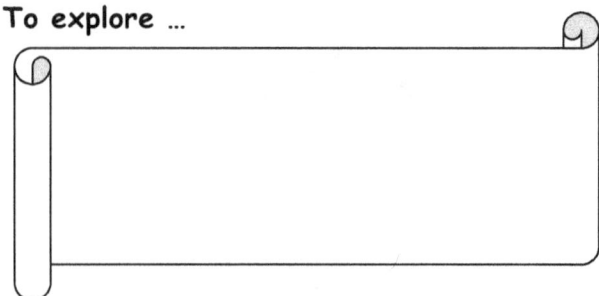

Energizing Idea 58:
Play outside.

"You can discover more about a person in an hour of play than in a year of conversation."
—Plato

Go play outside! Try swinging, sliding, hopping, skipping, jumping, climbing, biking, rolling, chasing, or any of your childhood favorites.

Play provides you with an opportunity to take risks. Play reduces stress, increases longevity, and stimulates imagination.

In 2011, Humana (a health care company) and KaBOOM (a nonprofit organization dedicated to promoting play for U.S. children) started building multigenerational playgrounds all over America. Grownups exercise on their own equipment while kids climb, dangle, and swing on theirs. There are stations for strengthening upper body/core, some for stretching/yoga postures, and others to increase mobility. These organizations got involved to fight obesity.

More inspiration:
- www.Humana.com
- www.KaBOOM.org
- www.HealthyMagination.com

Affirmation:
I love being playful!

Energizing Idea 59:
Control your portion size.

"Eat little, sleep sound."
—Iranian Proverb

Fast fact:
Americans often underestimate how many calories they are consuming each day by as much as 25 percent.

Do you have trouble knowing what your portion size should look like? You can use your hand as a quick guide to prevent overeating:

- About 1 cup = cupped hand (good for pasta, rice, beans, potatoes, cooked veggies, 1 oz. of nuts)
- About 1 cup = 2 hands cupped together (good for cereal, soup, casseroles, raw leafy veggies, salads)
- About 3 ounces = size and thickness of your palm (good for beef, poultry, fish)
- About 1 tablespoon = 2 thumbs together (good for salad dressing, peanut butter)
- About 1 teaspoon = thumb tip (oil, margarine, mayo, and "high fat" foods)
- Other: 1 tennis ball = about 1 serving of fruit

More inspiration:

- www.WebMd.com/diet/control-portion-size
- www.MeasureUpBowl.com (bowls with premeasured portions on their interior)

Affirmation:

I care for my body by watching the quantity of the foods I eat.

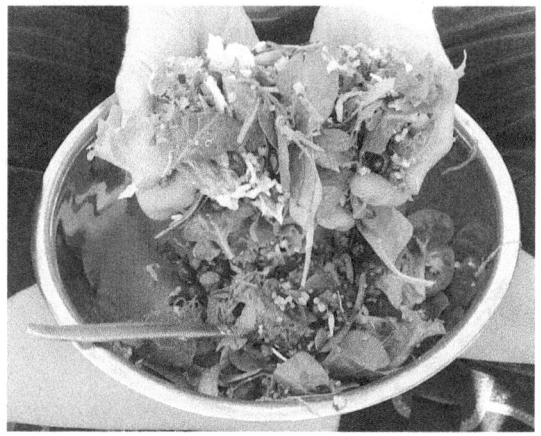

Energizing Idea 60:
Lose an excuse.

*"Excuses are the nails used
to build a house of failure."*
—Don Wilder

Write down your limiting excuses and beliefs.
Come face-to-face with these creative stories for
not living the life you want. You'll feel stronger.
You'll create space to grow and change. You are
what you believe.

Some common excuses:
- I'm too busy.
- I'm too tired.
- It's too risky.
- I can't afford it.
- I'm too old.
- I won't succeed.
- It can't be done.
- My friends/family wouldn't understand.

Do I have an excuse holding me back?
Where would I be without it?

_____

_____

More inspiration:
- *Excuses Begone! How to Change Lifelong Self-Defeating Thinking Habits* by Wayne Dyer
- *The 7 Habits of Highly Effective People: Powerful Lessons in Personal Change* by Stephen Covey

Affirmation:
Today I will overcome an old excuse, and
move forward.

Energizing Idea 61:
Unplug.

*"The excessive connectivity has created
false urgency."*
—Jay White

Every now and then, take a technology break.
Skip the e-mail and social media checks. Hide the
television remote. Leave the car keys on the hook.
It's okay!

What can I unplug?

_____

_____

_____

When?

_____

_____

_____

More inspiration:
- Your mind
- Your journal
- Your sketchpad

Affirmation:
Yippee … no gadgets! I feel great!

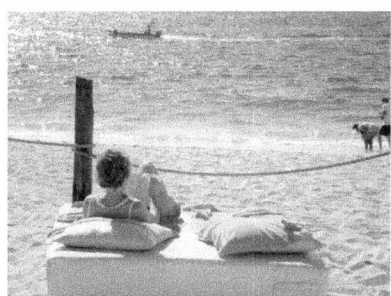

Cabo San Lucas, Mexico, April 2011

Energizing Idea 62:
Watch a sunrise or sunset.

*"There are only two ways to live your life.
One is as though nothing is a miracle. The
other is as though everything is a miracle."*
—Albert Einstein

Grab a jacket, hat, and gloves (if needed) and enjoy
a beautiful peaceful sunrise or sunset at the ocean,
on top of a mountain, or just outside your front
door. I love to hear the birds singing in my
neighbor's tree and feel the crisp morning air at
sunrise. I like to watch the sky's beauty at sunset
with a meditative walk. Whatever works for you is
just perfect.

More inspiration:
*   www.Weatherbug.com (sunrise, sunset times)
*   *Peace is Every Step* by Thich Nhat Hanh

Affirmation:
I take time to appreciate the world around me.
I feel nourished by this beautiful day.

Energizing Idea 63:
Dream big!

"Life is a great big canvas, and you should throw all the paint on it you can."
—Danny Kaye

You actually can be successful by believing you can. The "I believe I can" attitude sets the "can" and "how to" gears in motion. The energy you create gets the party started. The ideas you continue to generate, combined with action, keep it going.

More inspiration:
* *Think Big* by Ben Carson, M.D. with Cecil Murphey
* *The Magic of Thinking Big* by David J. Schwartz

Affirmation:
I am capable of anything my heart and mind can agree upon!

To explore ...

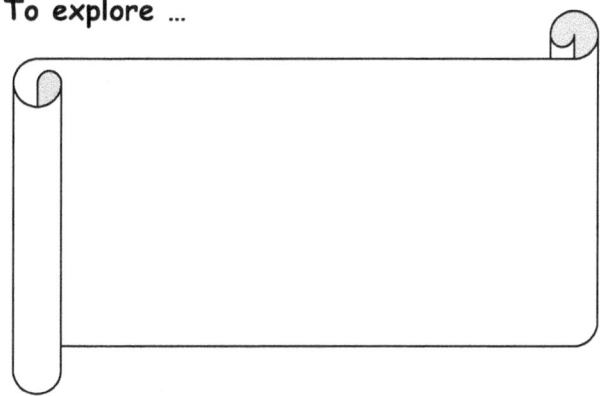

Energizing Idea 64:
Choose to be happy.

"Happiness is a perfume you cannot pour on others without getting a few drops on yourself."
—Ralph Waldo Emerson

"Happiness is like a butterfly; the more you chase it, the more it will elude you, but if you turn your attention to other things, it will come and sit softly on your shoulder."
—Henry David Thoreau

"A table, a chair, a bowl of fruit and a violin; what else does a man need to be happy?"
—Albert Einstein

Wild ideas on being happy!

_____

_____

More inspiration:
- Fabulous friends, music, and adventures
- *The 18 Rules of Happiness: How to be Happy* by Karl Moore
- *Enough Already: The Power of Radical Contentment* by Alan Cohen

Affirmation:
I choose to be happy. It looks good on me!

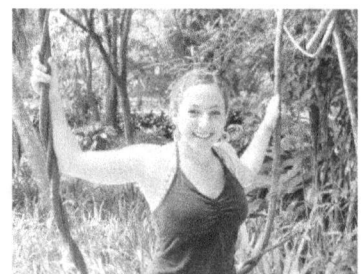

Happy Hillary in Brazil, June 2008

Energizing Idea 65:
Find out if you have a food allergy.

*"Food allergy affects an estimated 6 to 8
percent of children under age 5,
and about 3 to 4 percent of adults."*
—www.MayoClinic.com

A food allergy is an exaggerated immune response triggered by eggs, fish, peanuts, milk, or some other specific food. You might experience hives, blocked airways, wheezing, abdominal pain, itching, congestion, swelling, and/or other symptoms. If you have noticed an unpleasant reaction to eating certain food(s), consider getting tested for allergies.

More inspiration:
*   Allergy skin tests
*   Allergy elimination-type tests
*   Allergy blood tests
*   Your health provider

Affirmation:
I deserve to feel my best. I want to know what I am allergic to so I can avoid eating it.

To explore …

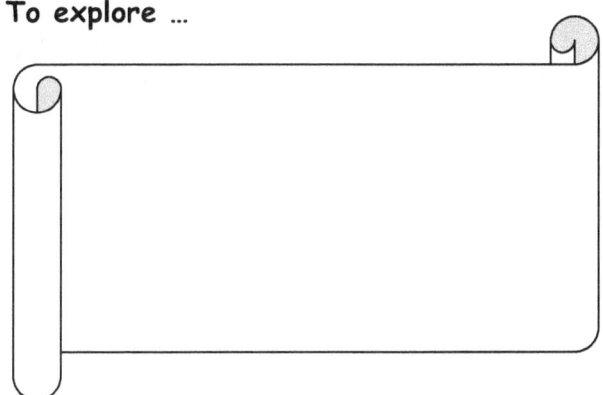

Energizing Idea 66:
Read, watch, or listen to
something inspirational.

*"Every great dream begins with a dreamer.
Always remember, you have within you
the strength, the patience, and the passion to
reach for the stars to change the world."*
—Harriet Tubman

Be inspired by great music, wise words of wisdom, fabulous art, beautiful performances, and so much more. How wonderful there are so many ways we can obtain (or share) inspiration!

More inspiration:
* *Inspiration: Your Ultimate Calling* by Wayne W. Dyer
* *The Book of Awakening: Having the Life You Want by Being Present to the Life You Have* by Mark Nepo

Affirmation:
I soak in the beauty, wisdom, and inspiration that is all around me.

To explore ...

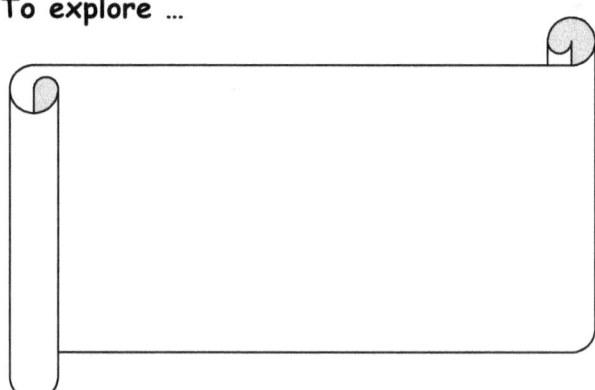

Energizing Idea 67:
Avoid being angry.

"Speak the truth. Give whatever you can. Never be angry. These three steps will lead you into the presence of the gods."
—Buddha

Save your energy and your need to apologize later! Develop strategies for dealing with people (and things) that make you angry.

Simple and effective techniques: Walk away, count to 10, breathe deeply, journal, talk to a loved one, or …

_____

_____

_____

More inspiration:

- *Transforming Anger: The Heartmath Solution for Letting Go of Rage, Frustration, and Irritation* by Doc Childre and Deborah Rozman
- www.apa.org/topics/anger/control.aspx

Affirmation:
For every minute I am angry, I lose 60 seconds of happiness.

Energizing Idea 68:
Eat low-glycemic foods
whenever possible.

"I recommend using the Glycemic Index as a guide to healthy carbohydrate consumption. In general, avoid frequent consumption and large servings of foods that rank high on this scale."
—Andrew Weil, M.D.

The Glycemic Index (GI) is a ranking of carbohydrates on a scale from 0 to 100 according to the extent to which they raise blood-sugar levels. It measures how much your blood glucose increases after eating.

0–54 = small rise in blood-sugar and insulin levels
55–70 = medium rise in blood-sugar and insulin levels
71–100 = fast rise in blood-sugar and insulin levels

Some examples of low and medium-glycemic foods: fruit, vegetables, beans, whole and multi-grain bread.

Examples of high-glycemic foods: candy, most cookies, white bread, soda, energy drinks, sugary cereals, and rice products.

Research shows low-GI foods can help control appetite, delay hunger, control weight, and prevent heart disease. They improve glucose and lipid levels in people with diabetes.

Eating high GI foods has many disadvantages:
- You receive a rush of energy, soon followed by an energy "crash."
- These foods increase your craving for sweeter foods.
- Your body uses this ineffective food source for energy, instead of tapping into your stored fat resources, making it harder to lose those extra pounds.

More inspiration:
- www.the-gi-diet.org
- *The G.I. Diet Express: For Busy People* by Rick Gallop

Affirmation:
I eat low-glycemic foods whenever I can. When I keep my blood-sugar levels steady, I feel great.

Energizing Idea 69:
Breathe deeply.

*"Fear less, hope more. Eat less, chew more.
Whine less, breathe more. Talk less,
say more. Love more, and all good things
will be yours."*
—Swedish proverb

Please take a deep breath. You have just added oxygen to every cell in your body!

I love how Thich Nhat Hanh encourages us to breathe "to make life vivid and more enjoyable." He says, "As you breathe in, you say to yourself, 'I know I am breathing in.' Just that. And as you breathe out, 'I know I am breathing out.' This technique can help you keep your mind on your breath."

More inspiration:
- Any Thich Nhat Hanh audio or book
- A yoga, Qigong, or meditation class
- Any Jon Kabat-Zinn audio or book

Affirmation:
I breathe deeply. I am alive and joyous.

Energizing Idea 70:
Live life with gusto!

"Whenever you go, go with all your heart."
—Confucius

Don Miguel Ruiz, author of *The Four Agreements,* reminds us to "always do your best."

He points out, "Your best is going to change from moment to moment. It will be different when you are healthy as opposed to sick. Under any circumstances, simply do your best and you will avoid self-abuse, and regret." He is a wise man!

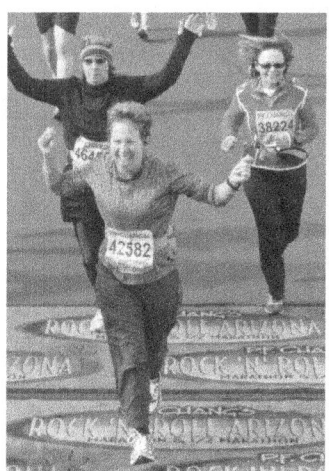

Phoenix, AZ, January 2007

More inspiration:
* *The Four Agreements* by Don Miguel Ruiz
* *Later Bloomers: 35 Folks Over Age 35 Who Found Their Passion and Purpose* by Debra Eve

Affirmation:
I enthusiastically give my all. I enjoy the blessings this practice brings me.

Energizing Idea 71:
As soon as you get up,
make your bed.

*"Especially if you're feeling overwhelmed,
picking one little task to improve your
situation, and doing it regularly, can help you
regain a sense of self-mastery. Making your
bed is a good place to start, and tackling an
easy daily step is a good way to energize
yourself for tougher situations."*
—Gretchen Rubin

Everyone is different. If making your bed doesn't work for you, perhaps there's another simple morning "ritual" that does work.

My energizing morning idea is …

_____
_____
_____

More inspiration:
- www.StevePavlina.com
- www.ZenHabits.net (a blog)

Affirmation:
I find energy in the little and the big tasks
I accomplish.

Energizing Idea 72:
Learn a new skill.
(Take a class, webinar, etc.)

"When I learn something new—
and it happens every day—I feel a little more
at home in this universe, a little more
comfortable in the nest."
—Bill Moyers

We're never too old to learn! Scientists have discovered adult brains are able to grow faster than previously thought. A few years ago, I did something really crazy. I took a four-credit anatomy class with my daughter. (Note: I had not stepped into a college classroom in more than 20 years!) It was the best thing I ever did for my brain!

More inspiration:
- *Learn Something Every Day* by Robert Young
- Online classes, colleges, community centers, books, magazines, other people, etc.

Affirmation:
Learning enhances my world, my mind, and my life.

To explore ...

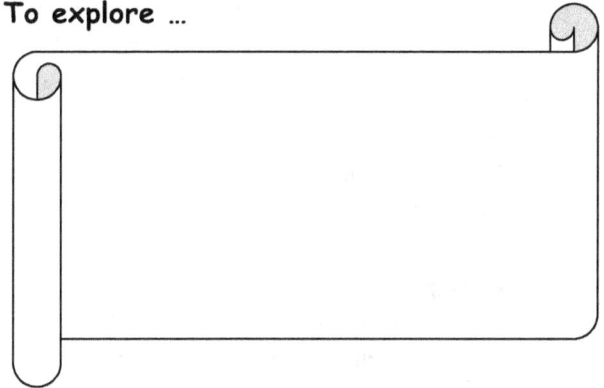

Energizing Idea 73:
Add some "zero calorie" foods to your meals.

"Elevate the quality of your food."
—Marc David

Although all foods contain calories, some foods take so much energy to digest that your body actually burns up the calories from them in the process of consuming them. These are called zero-calorie foods.

Zero-calorie foods: Apple, asparagus, beet, broccoli, cabbage, carrot, cauliflower, celery, chicory, cucumber, dandelion, endive, garden cress, garlic, grapefruit, green beans, hot chili pepper, lemon, lettuce, lime, mango, onion, orange, papaya, peach, pineapple, radishes, raspberries, spinach, strawberries, tangerine, tomato, turnip, zucchini

I love …

_____

_____

I'm going to try …

_____

_____

More inspiration:
- *The Essential Guide to Healthy Healing Foods* by JoAnn Milivojevic, Victoria Shanta Retelny
- www.WebMD.com/diet

Affirmation:
Zero-calorie fruits and vegetables are useful. They help control my weight while adding fiber and micronutrients to my meals.

Energizing Idea 74:
Remove junk food from your home, car, and office.

"If we're not willing to settle for junk living, we certainly shouldn't settle for junk food."
—Sally Edwards

Junk foods have little or no nutritional value. They often have ingredients unhealthy to eat. They are usually salty, sugary, and/or fried. I would put all sodas in the junk food category.

I recently read if we make our own healthy snack with just a little salt and just a little sweetness, we'll satisfy our cravings for junk food. My husband has created a perfect one for our at-home movie watching: air popped popcorn and apple slices ... add a bit of sea salt to the popcorn, if you like.

More inspiration:
*   *The Wholesome Junk Food Cookbook: More Than 100 Healthy Recipes for Everyday Snacking* by Laura Trice, M.D.
*   The healthy foods in your market

Affirmation:
I make it easier to maintain my healthy lifestyle by not keeping junk food around me.

To explore ...

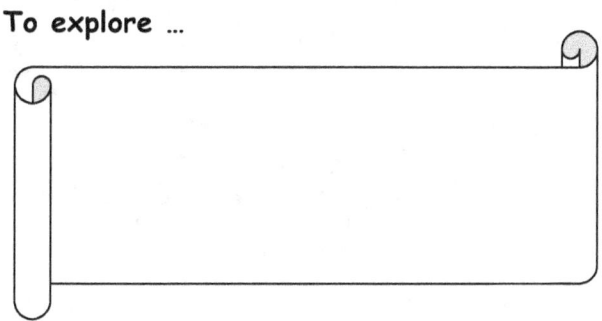

Energizing Idea 75:
Wear a fun scarf, silly socks, or both.

"Never put a sock in a toaster."
—Eddie Izzard

When I was a poor college student, my friends and I would give each other silly socks as gifts. Thirty years later, these dear women still bring adorable socks to our get-togethers. Love ya, Jeannie and Heidi!

How can you not feel energized while wearing silly socks, a bright scarf, or both? I'm so glad scarves are in!

More inspiration:
* Your local department store
* www.LittleMissMatched.com

Affirmation:
Dear friends and silly socks … what could be better!

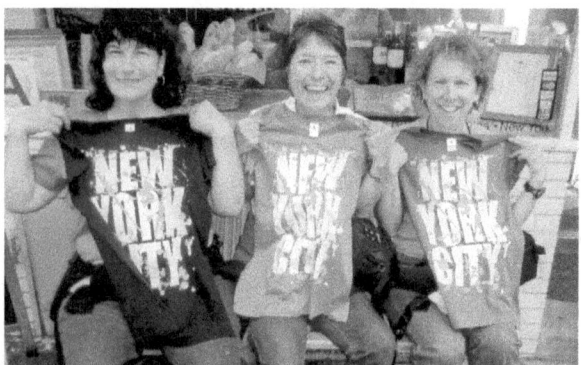

Heidi, Jeannie, and I in New York City,
October 2011

Energizing Idea 76:
Eat your legumes.

"Good things come in small packages."
—Author Unknown

Legumes (peas, beans, and lentils) are packed with top-quality protein, complex carbohydrates, fiber, vitamins, and minerals. Their ability to lower blood cholesterol helps to prevent heart disease. The slow way legumes are digested and absorbed makes them an ideal food for diabetics.

A delicious way to eat more beans is by making (or purchasing) hummus. It's fabulous as a salad-dressing substitute and as a dip for raw veggies. Here's a simple recipe:

Hummus
* 15-oz. can of garbanzo beans, drained
* 2/3 cup water (less for thicker hummus)
* 3 tablespoons tahini
* 1 large clove garlic
* ½ teaspoon salt
* 2 tablespoons olive oil
* 2 tablespoons lemon juice

Place all ingredients in a blender. Blend until creamy and serve. Refrigerate remaining hummus.

More inspiration:
* *More Easy Beans: Quick and Tasty Bean, Pea, and Lentil Recipes* by Trisha Ross, Jacquie Trafford
* www.SimpleDailyRecipes.com

Affirmation:
My body loves when I add legumes to my soups, salads, and dinner plate.

Energizing Idea 77:
Make peace with change.

"There is nothing permanent except change."
—Heraclitus

When we think of "change" it may bring up fear and other uncomfortable feelings. Remembering that things will change, because that's the way life works, makes it easier to deal with the process.

Here are some ideas that might help you make peace with change:

- Good or bad change? We don't know. It's too early to tell. Try not to hold tightly to the old. Embrace the new.

- Identify the changes you are going through. How do you feel? What lessons are being presented to you?

- Ask questions. Gather information. Be informed.

- Seek help if you need it.

- Overwhelmed? Break tasks down. Take action. Every step counts.

- Remind yourself you have done tougher things!

More inspiration:
- *Glad No Matter What: Transforming Loss and Change Into Gift and Opportunity* by SARK
- *Change Anything: The New Science of Personal Success* by Kerry Patterson, Joseph Grenny, David Maxfield, Ron McMillan, Al Switzler

Affirmation:
Change is inevitable. It's easier if I grab my boogie board and enjoy the waves.

Energizing Idea 78:
Get some sunlight.

*"I was a vegetarian until I started
leaning toward the sunlight."*
—Rita Rudner

- Our energy levels are linked to the cycle of the sun. We naturally have more energy during daylight.
- Getting 10 minutes of direct sun exposure each day helps the body produce Vitamin D. (But, please wear sunscreen while you are outside in the sun for extended periods of time.)
- Sunlight improves your digestion, elimination, and metabolism.
- Sunlight exposure encourages healthy circulation and enhances your immune system. It increases the oxygen in your blood.
- Getting enough sunlight during the day can help you sleep better at night.
- Sunlight helps to balance your hormones and lift your spirits.

More inspiration:
- *The Healing Sun: Sunlight and Health in the 21st Century* by Richard Hobday, Ph.D.
- *Winter Blues: Everything You Need to Know to Beat Seasonal Affective Disorder* by Norman E. Rosenthal, M.D.

Affirmation:
I love how sunlight makes me feel. I look forward to walking in the sun and feeling it on my face.

Energizing Idea 79:
Stretch.

"Everyone can learn to stretch, regardless of age or flexibility. You do not need to be in top physical condition or have specific athletic skills."
—Bob Anderson

Just by stretching, you can:
* Enhance energy and mood
* Reduce muscle tension
* Prevent injuries and make activities more enjoyable
* Increase range of movement
* Lower cholesterol (prolonged stretching)

More inspiration:
* *Stretching: 30th Anniversary Edition* by Bob Anderson
* *Full-Body Flexibility* – 2nd Edition by Jay Blahnik

Affirmation:
I freely give my body the gift of stretching. How lovely!

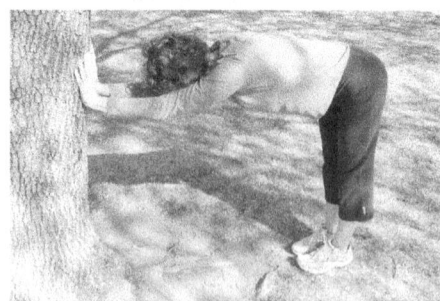

My favorite energy-booster stretch is a forward extension. Please keep your legs perpendicular to your upper body. Enjoy!

Energizing Idea 80:
Choose what is making you smile today.

"Sometimes your joy is the source of your smile, but sometimes your smile is the source of your joy."
—Thich Nhat Hanh

As we conclude our yoga class, my beautiful yoga teacher, Liisa asks, "What is making you smile today?" I absolutely love how this makes me feel… so do my classmates. See if stopping to answer this question helps you find a smile in your day.

Smiling is a fun way to live longer and happier.

More inspiration:
- *Smile For No Good Reason* by Lee L. Jampolsky
- Anything that helps you find a smile

Affirmation:
I pause throughout my day to ask, "What is making me smile today?" I share my smile with everyone I meet.

"You're never fully dressed without a smile."
—"Annie"

To explore …

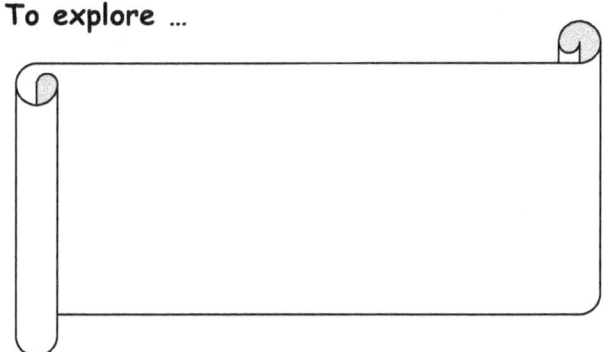

Energizing Idea 81:
Create a "survival kit" for a friend.

*"To the world you might be one person,
but to one person you might be the world."*
—Author Unknown

My friend Kae and I often exchanged "survival kits" before a trip, at the start of a new transition, or for no reason at all. I especially enjoyed the one she made for me just before I opened Bright Beginnings School. It included a copy of *Jonathan Livingston Seagull* by Richard Bach with many highlighted verses to remind me that I have no limits. Love you, Kae!

Share your wisdom and kindness by making a special survival kit for someone you hold dear. Include silly and sensible items sure to inspire creativity and laughter.

More inspiration:
- Your imagination
- A local bookstore, dollar store, thrift store, and card shop

Affirmation:
My friendships add so much joy to my life.

"Hold a true friend with both hands."
—African Proverb

Energizing Idea 82:
Take a mini-vacation.

"Oh, the places you'll go!"
—Dr. Seuss

Does it feel like everyone's going on vacation except you? You don't need to go far from home to add some zip to your step. Go on a mini-vacation ... a 1–3 day getaway that doesn't require tons of planning and doesn't cost a lot.

You'll recharge your batteries and get your mind off of work. Take a break from your regular routine. Maybe even catch some sunshine.

More inspiration:
- www.TripAdvisor.com
- www.Kayak.com
- Chamber of Commerce

Affirmation:
Mini-vacations recharge my batteries! I'm ready to go off to ...

_____

_____

_____

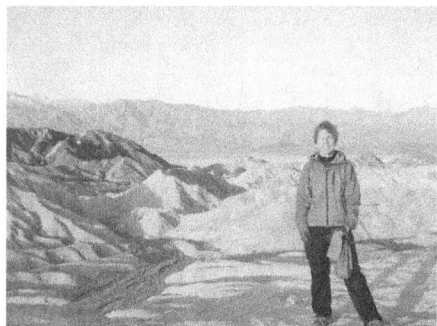

Death Valley National Park, California, February 2010

Energizing Idea 83:
Rub peppermint foot cream on your feet.

> *"If someone offers you a breath mint, accept it."*
> —H. Jackson Brown, Jr.

Aromatherapists have long relied on peppermint oil as a natural stimulant. Now scientists are on board. Researchers found that sniffing peppermint immediately improves both athletes' running speed and office workers' typing speed. The scent acts as a mood enhancer boosting your motivation and concentration. So grab an infusion—whether it's breath mints, lip gloss, hand lotion, or my favorite … foot cream.

More inspiration:
- Peppermint 100% pure essential oil
- Dr. Scholl's Cooling Peppermint Foot Lotion (inexpensive and invigorating)

Affirmation:
I treat myself to peppermint for a fabulous pick-me-up!

Energizing Idea 84:
Donate a bag of gently used clothing and household items to a local organization.

"If everybody in town donates one thread, a poor man has a shirt."
—African Proverb

Donating impacts lives. It helps families in need have a warm jacket, a comfortable blanket, shoes to walk to school, and so much more. Give what you can. Consider starting a collection box at your office. Donations are needed all year long.

More inspiration:
* Your local homeless shelter
* Big Brothers Big Sisters, www.bbbs.org

Affirmation:
I share my abundance with others in my community.

I'd like to make a difference by ...

_____
_____
_____
_____
_____

Energizing Idea 85:
Dance!

*"There are shortcuts to happiness
and dancing is one of them."*
—Vicki Baum

- Please do not overthink this one, friends. Turn your favorite music on and have fun dancing!
- Dancing tones your body, is great for your heart, offers protection against dementia, and frees your body to move without rules.
- Don't worry about how you look. Give yourself permission to have a good time.

More inspiration:

- If you love to dance, consider taking a class at your local community college or recreation center. Ask your friends for recommendations.
- Try an exercise class that involves dancing. Examples: Zumba or Nia

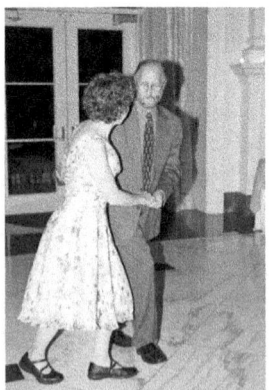

Dancing with my honey! November 2011

Affirmation:
Dancing makes me feel alive!

Energizing Idea 86:
Eat calcium-rich foods.

"Unless we constantly replenish our supply of calcium, drop by drop, our bones become thinner from depleting our calcium savings account. It's like living off your principal instead of your interest. It's not smart, and it puts you at risk for osteoporosis."
—Robert P. Heaney, M.D.

You already know calcium is crucial for building and maintaining healthy bones and teeth. Did you know it also plays an important role in the function of nerves, muscles, enzymes, and hormones? Spinach, watercress, parsley, dried figs, nuts, seeds, molasses, seaweed, and soy are all excellent suppliers of calcium.

Note:
Women who are postmenopausal are considered to be in a group at risk for calcium inadequacy, as decreases in estrogen production decreases calcium absorption.

More inspiration:
- National Institutes of Health: Office of Dietary Supplements
- Creighton University Osteoporosis Research Center

Affirmation:
I eat well to stay healthy and strong.

Energizing Idea 87:
Practice acts of kindness.

*"We make a living by what we get,
we make life by what we give."*
—Sir Winston Churchill

One of the best ways to energize your life is to help others. I like to do this in two ways:

1. On Wednesday afternoons, I volunteer. I help people over the age of 50 find employment.
2. I practice random acts of kindness. Each day this looks different. I might pick up trash, give a sandwich to a homeless person, help someone find his/her car at the mall, pay for a stranger's coffee, or leave fresh plums for a friend by her front door.

Whatever I do to help others brings me more energy and more joy than I ever imagined.

Be open to opportunities to help others.

My ideas for practicing kindness …

_____

_____

More inspiration:
*   www.RandomActsOfKindness.org
*   *The Power of Kindness: The Unexpected Benefits of Leading a Compassionate Life* by Piero Ferrucci

*"Do not wait for extraordinary circumstances
to do good; try to use ordinary situations."*
—Jean Paul Richter

Affirmation:
It is a joy to share kindness with those around me. I am so grateful to have the opportunity to help others.

Energizing Idea 88:
Eat fresh foods.

"My best nutritional advice: Avoid refined, processed, and manufactured foods."
—Dr. Andrew Weil

- Too much refined and processed food robs the body of vital nutrients and increases our intake of fat, sugar, and additives.
- Some of the most harmful ingredients in processed food include high-fructose corn syrup, trans fat, salt, artificial colors, and sweeteners.
- Due to heat in processing, canned fruits have a lower content of Vitamin C than fresh fruit.
- Several research studies suggest that eating processed meats may increase your risk for some types of cancer.

More inspiration:
- *The Eat Clean Diet for Family and Kids* by Tosca Reno
- Your favorite farmers' markets and other fresh-food markets

Affirmation:
Eating fresh food energizes my mind and body.

Energizing Idea 89:
Do the cross crawl.

"The cross crawl exercise reinforces the natural crossover of energy between the brain's left and right hemispheres, making learning easier. The cross crawl is also a great exercise whenever you feel lethargic and unmotivated."
—Gwenn Bonnell, based on the research of Paul and Gail Dennison

The cross crawl, named after the crawling movements of babies, is a wonderful quick exercise to energize your body. To try it, stand in place and lift the right knee to the left elbow. Return to standing. Now, lift the left knee to the right elbow. Repeat 5–10 times. (This exercise can be modified. It can be done sitting in a chair or lying down.)

It invigorates everyone regardless of age. Wise teachers have been using this exercise as a secret weapon for combating the 2 p.m. classroom slump for decades.

More inspiration:

*   *101 Great Ways to Improve Your Health,* selected and introduced by Dabid Riklan and Dr. Joseph Cilea. (101 mini-chapters, each written by a leading expert like Gwenn Bonnell)
*   *Brain Gym: Teacher's Edition* by Paul and Gail Dennison (26 activities to make learning easier)

Affirmation:

Kinesiology-based exercises are fun and energizing.
I'll add them to my bag of energy tricks!

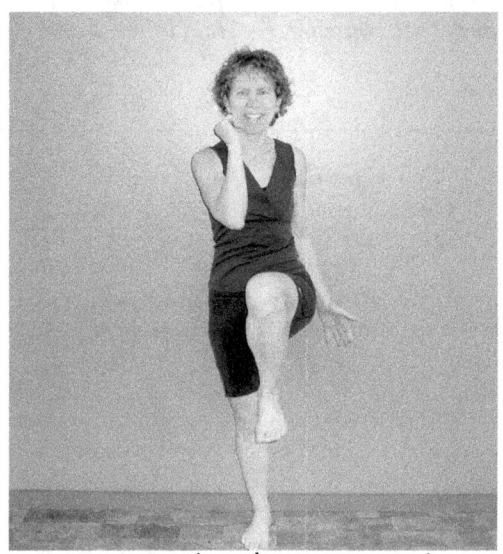

Demonstrating the cross crawl.

Energizing Idea 90:
Forgive for good.

*"Holding resentment is like eating poison
and then waiting for the other person
to keel over."*
—Unknown

"The Nine Steps to Forgiveness"
Created by Dr. Fred Luskin
Director of the Stanford Forgiveness Projects

1. Know exactly how you feel about what happened and be able to articulate what about the situation is not okay. Then tell a trusted couple of people about your experience.

2. Make a commitment to yourself to do what you have to do to feel better. Forgiveness is for you and not for anyone else.

3. Forgiveness does not necessarily mean reconciliation with the person who hurt you, or condoning of their action. What you are after is to find peace. Forgiveness can be defined as the "peace and understanding that come from blaming that which has hurt you less, taking the life experience less personally, and changing your grievance story."

4. Get the right perspective on what is happening. Recognize that your primary distress is coming from the hurt feelings, thoughts and physical upset you are suffering now, not what offended you or hurt you two minutes – or ten years – ago. Forgiveness helps to heal those hurt feelings.

5. At the moment you feel upset, practice a simple stress management technique to soothe your body's flight or fight response.

6. Give up expecting things from other people, or your life, that they do not choose to give you. Recognize the "unenforceable rules" you have for your health or how you or other people must behave. Remind yourself that you can hope for health, love, peace, and prosperity and work hard to get them.

7. Put your energy into looking for another way to get your positive goals met than through the experience that has hurt you. Instead of mentally replaying your hurt, seek out new ways to get what you want.

8. Remember that a life well lived is your best revenge. Instead of focusing on your wounded feelings, and thereby giving the person who caused you pain power over you, learn to look for love, beauty and kindness around you. Forgiveness is about personal power.

9. Amend your grievance story to remind you of the heroic choice to forgive.

The practice of forgiveness has been shown to reduce anger, hurt, depression and stress. It leads to greater feelings of hope, peace, compassion, and self-confidence. Practicing forgiveness leads to healthy relationships as well as physical health. It also influences our attitude, which opens the heart to kindness, beauty, and love.

More inspiration:
- www.LearningToForgive.com
  (Dr. Fred Luskin's website)
- *How Can I Forgive You? The Courage to Forgive, the Freedom Not To* by Janis A. Spring

Affirmation:
Practicing forgiveness opens my heart to beauty, kindness, and love.

Energizing Idea 91:
Open your body's energy flow
with Qigong.

*"Qigong is an ancient Chinese exercise form
that retards the aging process by cultivating
and strengthening vital energy in the body."*
—Shoshanna Katzman

Qigong (pronounced chee-GUNG) is a practice
involving flowing postures. These movements are
slow and circular.

Qigong is a lovely blend of regulated breathing,
focused meditation, and self-massage. There are
many styles; some gentler like tai chi, others more
vigorous like kung fu.

Benefits:
- Greater stamina and vitality
- Lower blood pressure
- Reduced stress
- Better balance
- Enhanced immune system
- Improved digestion

More inspiration:

- *Practice Easy Tai Chi–Qi Gong with Kim Kubsch,* a terrific 45-minute DVD available at www.SafeMovements.com
- *Qigong for Staying Young: A Simple 20-Minute Workout to Cultivate Your Vital Energy* by Shoshanna Katzman

Affirmation:

Qigong is a gentle and effortless way to move. There are so many benefits … I will try it!

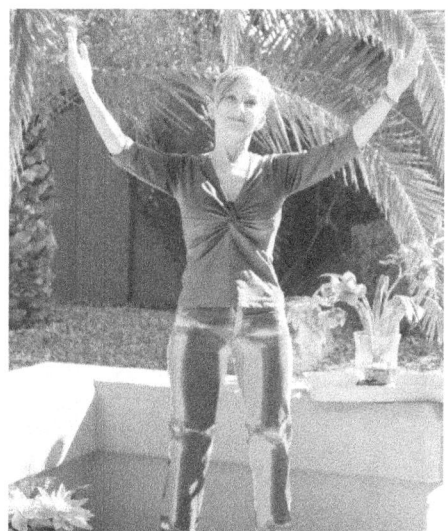

Kim Kubsch teaching Qigong.

Energizing Idea 92:
Walk in the rain.

"Everyone wants happiness, no one wants pain, but you can't make a rainbow without a little rain."
—Author Unknown

Many people believe a rainy day means staying indoors and waiting for the sun to shine again. There are other people who love to walk in the rain.

My lovely daughter, Hillary, never seems bothered by a rainy day. She doesn't modify her plans and doesn't let her mood change. I admire her amazing go-with-the-flow upbeat attitude.

Marian Marbury, the CEO of Adventures in Good Company, says there is no bad weather, only bad gear. She's so much fun to travel with!

More inspiration:
*   www.AdventuresInGoodCompany.com
    (best adventure travel for women)
*   www.REI.com
    (my favorite place to buy rain wear)

Affirmation:
I'm singing in the rain!

Energizing Idea 93:
Join a group.

"I don't care to belong to a club that accepts people like me as members."
—Groucho Marx

Networking groups. Social-media groups. Fitness groups. Special-interest groups. Getting involved in a group can be beneficial in many ways. You can learn more about a particular topic, make some new friends, find an accountability partner, increase your potential business contacts, and so much more.

I love my networking groups and hiking groups. I enjoy being around kind, warm, like-minded people who want to have fun.

More inspiration:
* www.MeetUp.com
* www.Groups.Google.com
* www.LinkedIn.com

Affirmation:
I enjoy socializing, networking, and being around terrific people.

To explore ...

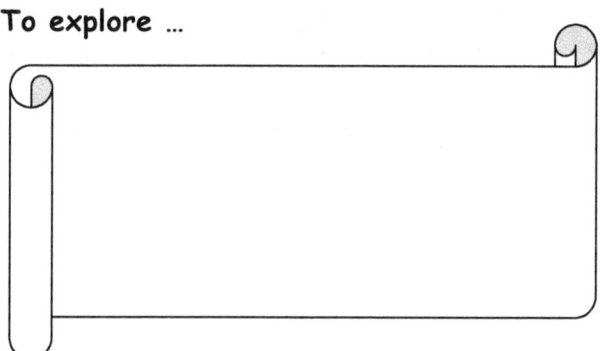

Energizing Idea 94:
Go on a picnic.

"If ants are such busy workers, how come they find time to go to all the picnics?"
—Marie Dressler

Ellen's Corner Picnic Blog
January 28, 2010
www.PicnicSupplyWorld.com

When we hear some words, they connect us with pleasure, play, etc. One such word that brings us close to our happiness is "picnic." The moment we hear or overhear the word "picnic" it takes us to a new feeling of joy.

I want to let you know the benefits that a picnic can bring us. Though it appears to be a casual event, it has huge advantages associated with it, directly and indirectly.

Bonding: A picnic connects all the members to have an understanding about each other. As people find it hard to bond on normal days, a picnic provides a perfect place to associate with the family, co-workers, or even superiors.

Fun: Picnics are fun events. Many of us are stressed out with monotonous work or vexed with a challenging relationship, or even bored doing mundane tasks. A picnic acts as a change agent and adds a touch of life, rejuvenating us holistically.

Beauty: A picnic usually happens in the lap of nature, thus bringing us closer to its serenity and awesome beauty. Nature itself acts as an open health spa by allowing us to breathe fresh air and generates a feeling of euphoria.

Team spirit: Most picnics are loaded with fun games. Playing with new people allows us to develop team spirit. Each one contributes his part to make his team win. We work for a common goal and this indirectly makes us feel good.

Network: A picnic is a gathering of diverse individuals. You may find a mentor to guide, a friend for life, or even your future life partner on such occasions. It is a great platform to find people who interest you. Relationships flourish, naturally.

More inspiration:
* www.PicnicSupplyWorld.com

Affirmation:
I look forward to grabbing an old blanket, a picnic lunch, and my buddies ... let's go on a picnic!

Energizing Idea 95:
Sign up for free
motivational quotes.

"Inspiration and genius—one and the same."
—Victor Hugo

- I have received free quotes from www.TaroGold.com for many years. Always great.
- Alan Cohen has free quotes and a lovely monthly newsletter. To receive his quotes, go to www.AlanCohen.com.
- Open your e-mail quotes and add a lift to your spirit.

More inspiration:
- www.UpliftingIdeas.com
- www.Inspirational-Quotes.info

Affirmation:
A dose of daily inspiration is like a breath of fresh air. I enjoy the words of wisdom I receive.

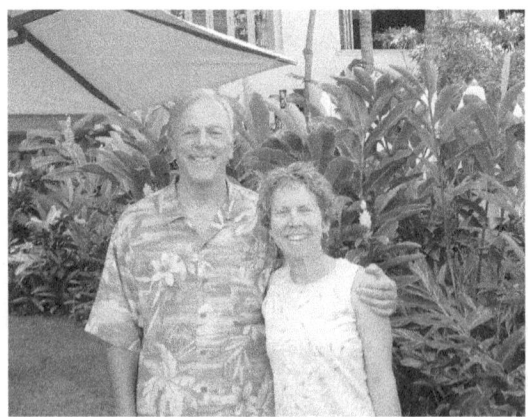

Alan Cohen and I, December 2010
I had the privilege of hearing Alan speak in
Maui. He was terrific!

Energizing Idea 96:
Soak up compliments.

*"I can live for two months
on a good compliment."*
—Mark Twain

Many of us have difficulty accepting compliments and grateful comments. We often react with embarrassment or minimize the compliment. For example, when we are thanked for something done well, some respond, "Oh, that was nothing!"

Instead of responding with a quick "thank you," take a moment to let the compliment seep into every pore. This will energize both you and the giver.

More inspiration:
*   www.WikiHow.com/Take-Compliments
*   *The Compliment Quotient: Boost Your Spirits, Spark Your Relationships and Uplift Your World* by Monica Strobel

Affirmation:
I am worthy of receiving praise, compliments, and all the richness life has to offer.

To explore ...

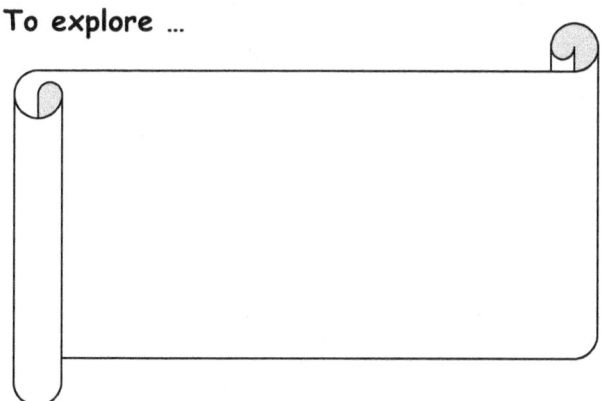

Energizing Idea 97:
De-clutter for 10 minutes.

"Lost time is never found again."
—Benjamin Franklin

Clutter can fill the smooth day-to-day moments of your life with added stress and zap your energy. Where are those keys? That phone number? When you're staring at a stack of papers and piles of stuff, beginning to de-clutter may seem overwhelming.

Here are two energizing ideas to get you started:

1. Schedule 10 minutes to tackle a specific de-cluttering project. If it's not complete, schedule another 10-minute block. Enjoy the progress you made without beating yourself up for not completing the task.

2. Resolve to try Gretchen Rubin's "One-Minute Rule:" If a task can be done in less than a minute, go for it ... right then and there! (Example: hang up your sweater when you come home, take out garbage, etc.)

Areas I give myself permission to de-clutter for blocks of 10 minutes ...

_____

_____

_____

_____

_____

More inspiration:

- www.Unclutter.com
- www.GretchenRubin.com

Affirmation:

As I de-clutter my life, I make room for special treasures to come in.

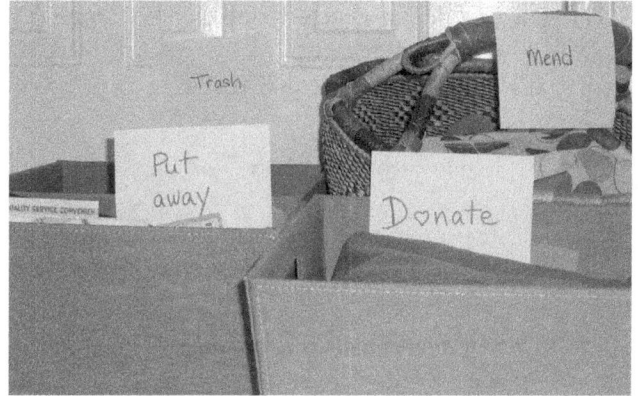

Energizing Idea 98:
Have some chocolate protein pudding!

"Life is like a box chocolates ... you never know what you're gonna get."
—Forrest Gump (played by Tom Hanks)

Here is a protein-packed snack the whole family will love for many reasons:

• It's quick to prepare.

• It's sweet.

• It's low in carbs and sugar.

Chocolate protein pudding (1 generous serving):

• 6 ounces of plain unsweetened yogurt (Greek, soy, etc.)*

• 1 scoop high-quality chocolate protein powder

• Stevia natural sweetener (optional)

* My favorite yogurt is "cultured coconut milk" made by So Delicious. It's dairy-free, soy-free, and tastes amazing!

Directions:
1. In a small bowl, combine the yogurt and protein powder. Stir until all lumps have disappeared.
2. Add Stevia, if you desire.

Affirmation:
It's fun to take an old favorite snack and make it healthier.

Energizing Idea 99:
I am the kind of person who ...

_____

_____

"It's never too late to be what you
might have been."
—George Eliot

Instead of creating New Year's resolutions,
every couple of months try completing the
above sentence with a new small obtainable goal.
No pressure. Have fun. Get energized! (You don't
have to be perfect!)

My current one is: "I am the kind of person who
shows up early without rushing." I am loving the
new me ... the lady who leaves more time to get to
appointments, arrives early for fitness classes, lunch
dates, etc. (If I arrive "too early," I read, journal, or
enjoy breathing in the peacefulness.)

More inspiration:
- Your journal. Your wild ideas!
- Your Vision Board
- "Who have you come here to be?"
  (inspirational card deck from
  www.TheQEffect.com)

Sample affirmations:
I am the kind of person who eats healthy food.
I am the kind of person who keeps fit. I am the
kind of person who maintains a good body weight.

My affirmation:

_____

_____

Energizing Idea 100:
Begin.

*"Whatever you do, or dream you can,
begin it. Boldness has genius power,
and magic in it."*
—Johann Wolfgang von Goethe

The first step to starting a new project is often the hardest. It takes courage and guts, but the results are energizing! So just begin ... you may stumble, you may not have the most graceful beginning but once you get started the creative juices will flow and you'll be glad you did. Don't overthink it.

More inspiration:
- Inspirational magazines or books in your field
- Webinars in your field

Affirmation:
I embrace beginnings and all they inspire.

To explore ...

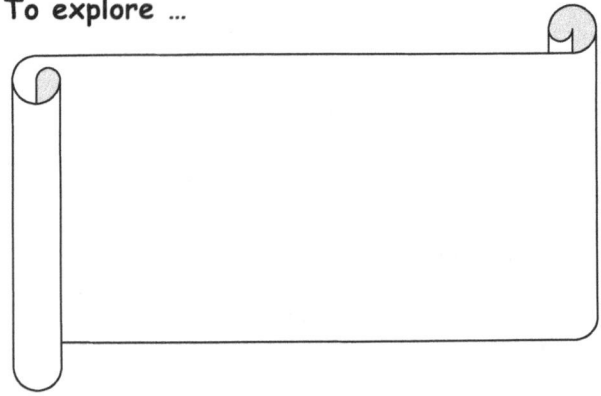

My Energizing Idea 101:

_____
_____

My quote ...

_____
_____
_____

My wisdom ...

_____
_____
_____

My resource(s) ...

_____
_____
_____

My affirmation ...

_____
_____
_____

To explore ...

_____
_____
_____

My photo or drawing ...

Today, I will have a go at ...

- Energizing Idea #_____
- Energizing Idea #_____
- Energizing Idea #_____
- Energizing Idea #_____
- Energizing Idea #_____
-
-
-
-
-

Soon, I will have a go at ...

- Energizing Idea #_____
- Energizing Idea #_____
- Energizing Idea #_____
- Energizing Idea #_____
- Energizing Idea #_____
-
-
-
-
-

Acknowledgements

*"Some people are so much sunshine
to the square inch."*
—Walt Whitman

With heaps of gratitude for:

- The students I have taught in my three decades as an educator. I have learned so much from you. xo.

- My colleagues from Bright Beginnings School. It's such a joy to have you in my life. What an incredible school we created from a big dirt lot! xo.

- Brandi Walsh and Katrina Joyner, my talented artists at DoneWellDesign.com and SpearCarrier.daPortfolio.com. xo.

- Ann Videan, my splendid editor and long-time friend. Thanks for your amazing eyes, terrific mind, and warm heart. xo.

- Heidi, Jeannie, Nadine, and Sue. We have been dear friends for more than 40 years! (How can this be possible?) xo.

- Energetic Jeri, Joyful Janet, Merry Mary, and Wild Sandra, my adventure buddies. Thanks for sharing trail mix and kindness. xo.

- My "families" at Fitness Forum and Sol Yoga … the people who see me without makeup, often before the sun even thinks of rising. You are my morning cup of sweetness! xo.

- Adabelle, Kim, Liisa, Patty, and Stephanie. You keep me balanced, fit, and sane. It takes five woman to do this…oh my! xo.

- The Hoffman and Falk extended families. You're the best! xo.

- Marvelous Uncle Morry. You are such a special light in my life. xo.

- Delightful Daniel, my incredible honey. Thanks for believing in me even when I don't. Your unconditional love fuels my day. I love you wholeheartedly. Book's done ... let's go dancing! xo.
- Awesome Hillary, my amazing daughter. Thanks for choosing me to be your mom; I'm honored. Love you from here to the Sun and back. I am so proud of you! xo.

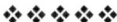

"Nothing is as powerful as an idea whose time has come—and you are that idea."
—Alan Cohen

> There are so many additional brilliant ways to energize our day. I'd love to hear your favorite idea ... that thing you do to bring a zip to your step and a twinkle to your eye!
>
> I look forward to gathering your energizing tips and photos together for *More All-Day Energy!* Each published idea will have your name, hometown, and website link. Thanks so much for sharing!
>
> With peace, joy, gratitude, and love,
>
> Syd
> Syd@SydHoffman.com

About Syd

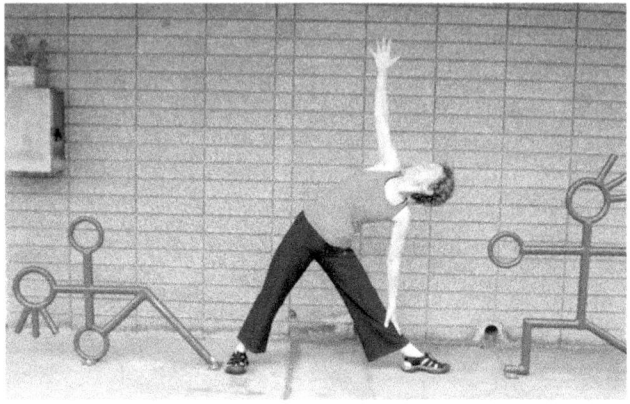

Health and wellness expert Syd Hoffman is a speaker, author, and coach. She has motivated and inspired people on five continents to create a lifetime of healthy living, one step at a time. She loves sharing her passion for healthy living on radio and television, and in person. Her seminars, workshops, retreats, and "one-on-one lifestyle tweaks" will energize your life.

Syd started lifting weights, setting her elliptical to an insane grade, and practicing yoga all *after* the age of 40. It took her almost five years to comfortably touch her toes and she learned a lot about herself on the journey. A balanced fitness program with six healthy meals a day keeps this very busy lady smiling all day long!

A talented entrepreneur, Syd created and sold two very successful businesses: an elementary school and a fitness center. She is a lifelong learner and teacher who firmly believes life is best when we eat well, play hard, and hug often. She really, really, *really* enjoys hiking tall mountains in faraway places, a slow run, practicing yoga on a mat right next to her incredible daughter, and her newest hobby … Lindy Hop dancing with her dreamy husband.

Please visit www.SydHoffman.com to learn more secrets of high-energy people and to find future events: presentations, videos, seminars, retreats, and Syd's All-Day Energy Summits!

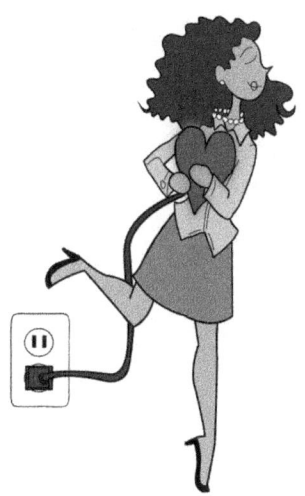

www.ingramcontent.com/pod-product-compliance
Lightning Source LLC
Chambersburg PA
CBHW070148290526
45789CB00002B/682